UNDERSTAND HOW TO

REST AND RECOVER IN THIS "ALWAYS ON" SOCIETY

TAKE BACK YOUR TIME TO REST AND UNWIND
AND BECOME A BETTER VERSION OF YOURSELF

JESSIE FIELDS

Copyright © 2022 by Shopsterise Ltd - All rights reserved.

The contents of this book may not be reproduced, duplicated or transmitted without direct written permission from the author.

Under no circumstances will any legal responsibility or blame be held against the publisher for any reparation, damages, or monetary loss due to the information herein, either directly or indirectly.

Legal Notice:

This book is copyright protected. This is only for personal use. You cannot amend, distribute, sell, use, quote or paraphrase any part or the content within this book without the consent of the author.

Disclaimer Notice:

Please note the information contained within this document is for educational and entertainment purposes only. Every attempt has been made to provide accurate, up to date, and reliable complete information. No warranties of any kind are expressed or implied. Readers acknowledge that the author is not engaging in the rendering of legal, financial, medical or professional advice. The content of this book has been derived from various sources. Please consult a licensed professional before attempting any techniques outlined in this book.

By reading this document, the reader agrees that under no circumstances is the author responsible for any losses, direct or indirect, which are incurred as a result of the use of the information contained within this document, including, but not limited to,
—errors, omissions, or inaccuracies.

Contents

Introduction 1

1. Defining Rest 3
2. Why is rest important? 17
3. What happens if we don't get enough rest? ... 31
4. Sleep 47
5. Exercise 57
6. The relaxing power of a hobby 69
7. Meditation and Mindfulness 83
8. Forest bathing and the healing power of nature ... 95
9. Breathing - Take a deep breath 107

Conclusion 117

Introduction

Do you feel as if you never have enough time in your day to rest? Do you constantly forget things or feel like you are always playing catch up? Then you have picked up the right book!

After reading this book, you'll understand what defines good rest, why rest is so important, the health benefits of good rest, and strategies for implementing more rest into your life.

In the first few chapters of the book, we'll define the idea of rest and explore the different types of rest. Next, we'll cover why rest is essential to our psychological, physical, and mental health. Finally, we'll also look into the consequences of not getting enough rest for our health and well-being. These first chapters will build a foundation of knowledge and help us understand why rest is so essential for us to function at our best.

But how can we relax and unwind after a busy day? The following chapters will discuss common problems we face concerning rest and offer tips and solutions. First, we'll discuss sleep, how it differs from rest, and what defines good quality sleep. We'll also look into different sleep disorders and strategies for getting good sleep. Next, the topic of exercise will be explored, and we'll gain an understanding of the specific recommendations for various age groups. We'll also discover the importance of hobbies. We will cover how to find a new hobby, why having a hobby is essential, the health benefits of having a hobby, and what differentiates a "hobby" from an "interest".

Finally, we'll look into meditation and mindfulness, breathing, and ecopsychology (emphasizing forest bathing). These techniques can be excellent ways to switch off and unwind. There are plenty of apps (both free and paid options) to help with guided meditation and breathing exercises in today's digital age, making this very accessible and affordable for anyone.

Why is it so difficult for us to get enough rest? By understanding our modern history and our ancestral roots, we'll learn more about why we struggle so much these days to get the rest we need. Throughout the book, we'll examine this within the context of our current society and digital technology's impact on our needs and challenges.

Although this book is based on the latest scientific studies and can be viewed as a synopsis of these (a citation reference can be found at the end of the book), it also includes advanced scenarios and tips you can implement in real-life. However, this book is not meant to replace a mental health professional. If you find yourself struggling, experience extreme distress or anxiety, or are experiencing any other mental health issue, please reach out to a trained mental health professional for assistance.

So, are you ready to learn more about the importance of rest and how to make sure you get enough of it? Read on!

Chapter One

Defining Rest

Brina is a 34-year-old businesswoman with a high-stress job at a university. She finds herself constantly thinking about work, so much so that it is beginning to interfere with other parts of her life. Working from home has made the situation even worse, and lately, she's had a lot of trouble "switching off" at the end of the day. Brina finds herself picking up her phone and refreshing her emails during dinner to ensure there aren't any fires that need immediate attention. She often wakes up before her alarm and checks her emails before even getting out of bed. Her husband has started making comments that he is worried about her, but she's assured him it isn't forever and that this is temporary until her new team is fully hired and onboarded.

Brina often finds herself working well beyond her scheduled hours, which causes her to struggle to balance her work and home life. She sneaks a peek at her phone while she's supposed to be watching her son kick field goals, and sometimes she feels like a terrible parent. She's drowning in responsibilities, and all she really wants is some rejuvenating rest.

Does any of this sound familiar to you? If so, you have picked up the right book, as we will now learn about stress and the importance of good rest.

To define rest, we first should address what stress is.

What is stress?

"Stress is the feeling of being overwhelmed or unable to cope with mental or emotional pressure" ("Stress", 2021, para 1).

Stress can come from different places, such as work, family issues, financial strains, relationships, or personal trauma. In Brina's case, most of her stress stems from her job responsibilities and the struggle to maintain a work-life balance. Stress can manifest in many different ways. For Brina, stress looks like a racing heartbeat and intrusive thoughts. Mentally, one might feel anxious, depressed, or overwhelmed. Physically, stress can manifest as increased heart rate, high blood pressure, headaches, and many other symptoms. Socially, people may withdraw from their friends and family or become irritable and frustrated with those they love. In the long term, stress can be physically harmful to our bodies and lead to certain illnesses, such as IBS, cardiovascular disease, and stomach ulcers.

So how can we reduce stress in a world that equates work with success and glorifies the never-ending "hustle culture"? The answer is rest.

What is rest?

Defining rest is difficult. The most straightforward definition is "the cessation of activity", although this does not address the many complexities that our society is faced with today. What constitutes activity? What is the threshold for cessation? Academics have attempted to define rest through various lenses:

- In healthcare, rest can be defined by measuring heart rate and blood pressure. Patients who need rest should be inactive, comfortable, and have "minimal functional and metabolic activity". This rest is essential for patients who have recently undergone surgery as it allows them to regain strength and heal properly.

- In spirituality, rest is defined as tranquility, peace of mind or spirit, calmness, or a feeling of "being at home" in one's body and mind. In Eastern religions, meditation is an integral part of rest and allows people to build new resources.

- Physiologically speaking, rest is the basis of Maslow's hierarchy of needs, where rest forms the basic, foundational building block of well-being and health. Rest affects many bodily functions such as circadian rhythms, hormone production, and metabolism. The concept of "stillness" is also included under this umbrella.

Types of rest

Mental Rest

Our brains are constantly under stress throughout the day, as we take in a variety of information from many different sources and try to respond accordingly. From choosing what to eat for lunch to answering emails, our brains are continuously transitioning between tasks.

Being mindful of what causes our stress is vital to figuring out the best strategies for addressing it. An excellent way to understand this stress is journaling. According to Holstee (n.d.), the benefits of journaling include:

- Reduction of anxiety and depression – Journaling allows us to address psychological issues that interfere with our mental rest. It has been shown to help with anxiety, depression, and many other psychological problems. Studies have also shown that journaling can help with "intrusive" thoughts, which are persistent and usually harmful or detrimental in some way. In our previous example, Brina suffers from intrusive thoughts about work. These thoughts plague her while she is involved in unrelated activities like watching her son's game. She cannot stop these thoughts from interrupting her throughout the day. We can get the thoughts out of our heads and onto paper through journaling. This detachment from our thoughts can help us view patterns and solve problems more objectively.

- Cultivating gratitude – By drawing attention to the many positive things we have in our lives, we can boost our gratitude and optimism and become more pleasant and friendly. Gratitude allows us to take stock of the good in our lives, focus less on the negatives, and thus achieve mental rest more easily. The more we practice cultivating gratitude, the easier it becomes to integrate it into our mental framework.

- Trauma Recovery – Most of us have faced some trauma in our lives. When trauma is unresolved in our minds, we cannot stop focusing on it, resulting in us being unable to rest mentally. Journaling allows us to confront our experiences rather than avoid them, so we can process them and move on in a healthy way. When we can effectively distance ourselves from these events, we can allow more space for mental health and rest.

- Improved Memory Function – Journaling can boost long-term memory, illuminate patterns, and allow us to reflect on ourselves. By addressing unhealthy habits we may perpetuate, we can then change our behaviors (both mentally and physically) to promote more rest in our lives.

Physical Rest

Our bodies need physical rest even if we don't have particularly physically demanding jobs. For example, those of us who work in offices can face issues with eye strain, posture, neck pain, and many other ailments that come from sitting and staring at a computer for many hours.

The field of Ergonomics studies the relationship between people, their bodies, and efficacy in the workplace. These studies ultimately affect how products are designed to promote safe and effective workplaces. Ergonomics is important to consider when thinking about ways to help our bodies rest. In the office, things like desk design, keyboard height, and chair type are all important considerations when thinking about how well our bodies work. Poor ergonomics can lead to bad posture and other injuries such as carpal tunnel syndrome. Repetitive motions are also required in many different types of jobs, which can lead to injury. When these issues are addressed, our bodies can have an easier time resting. Many large companies and businesses may have Ergonomists on-site to assist with these issues. Federal industries may work closely with Occupational Safety and Health Administration (OSHA) to ensure worker safety. When we put physical safety nets in place at our workplaces, we avoid undue strain on our bodies which can have long-term effects that interfere with well-being (Roth, 2011).

When thinking about physical rest, one part of our bodies that is often overlooked (no pun intended) is our eyes. Those who work on a computer all day may be vulnerable to eye strain. In the digital age, a common ailment is Computer Vision Syndrome (CVS), where people may experience eye dryness, headaches, shoulder and neck pain, and even blurred vision. This syndrome is caused by poor lighting (either within the office or emanating from the computer), having the computer too close or too far away, and screen glare.

Some ways to address CVS include anti-glare screens, frequent blinking, proper lighting, and the appropriate location of the screen itself (15-20 degrees below eye level and 20-28 inches or 50-70 cm away from the eyes). An easy rule to remember to help rest our eyes is the 20-20-20 Rule; for every 20 minutes spent looking at a screen, you should look at something 20 feet (6 meters) away for 20 seconds (Nall, 2019).

Specific hobbies can also tax our eyes. For example, for those who enjoy reading in the evening, it's essential to consider its effect on us. E-Readers such as the Kindle and Nook have risen in popularity in the digital age. This rise has again caused some concerns among the scientific community. Although not many studies have been done on this issue, results suggest that LCD eReaders (such as the Kindle Fire HD) trigger more visual fatigue than E-ink readers (such as the Kindle Paperwhite). This visual fatigue could be due to the way these devices are lit. LCD eReaders work by emitting light through their display and directly towards the eyes (similar to how smartphones work). In contrast, E-ink devices are considered "reflective displays", and no backlight is used.

Additionally, considerations regarding traditional paperback books should be taken into account. When reading traditional books, the quality of light is essential. Poor lighting makes focusing more difficult, which leads to less blinking and dryer eyes. Reading a traditional book in the dark with a book light may be kinder to the eyes than an E-Reader because the light reflects off the book's pages instead of shining directly into the eyes (The Best of Health, 2020).

Overall, it's vital to think about our whole bodies regarding physical rest. Even those often overlooked parts.

Spiritual Rest

Spiritual rest can include reconnecting with your spiritual community through attending worship services, local events, or community service. This type of rest can also involve a form of mindfulness through the readings of religious or spiritual texts and connecting to personal values to find meaning.

In our current culture, some religious groups have integrated technological dependence into their ideas of rest. For example, in Los Angeles, a Jewish group called "Reboot" organized a "National Day of Unplugging" to tie traditional Jewish customs to our current hectic lives in the Digital Age. The organization created a Sabbath Manifesto (in the Jewish tradition, the Sabbath is a day of rest) that can be utilized by any religion or by those with no religious affiliation at all. The manifesto, a new take on the Sabbath tradition, asks participants to "avoid technology, connect with loved ones, nurture your health, get outside, avoid commerce, light candles, drink wine, eat bread, find silence and give back" (Morris, 2011).

The benefits of modern religious tradition are interesting to consider, even for those not involved in organized religion. The ideas of spirituality and religion can also be separated. Mindfulness and meditation stem from Buddhist practice and will be further covered later in this book.

Sensory Rest

According to Guttman (2019), sensory rest is essential in order to avoid sensory overload, which can produce physiological effects, such as increased heart rate and blood pressure, and pronounced irritability and confusion. Sensory overload is considered overstimulation of our senses. It can be caused by clutter, multitasking, and technology overuse.

Physical sensory overload can occur when an environment contains too much clutter or too many objects. Scientific studies have shown that clutter can substantially impact mood and self-esteem and even produce increased cortisol levels (the stress hormone). There are many different strategies for reducing physical clutter. While not always enjoyable, tidying up can help our bodies relax in their environment.

Psychological sensory overload can occur when we overwhelm ourselves with too much stimulation, be it social, technological, or otherwise. This type of overload can induce an unwarranted "fight or flight" response in us and cause our brains to work less efficiently. Techniques for reducing psychological sensory overload include meditation (addressed more in Chapter 7) and reducing technology use.

**If you find yourself struggling to remove physical clutter, experience extreme distress or anxiety when thinking about clearing clutter, or find yourself in an unsafe physical space due to your clutter, please reach out to a trained mental health professional for assistance.

Creative Rest

Creativity can be defined as the action of making a novel work or product that did not exist previously in precisely the same form. Creativity looks different for everyone and can include activities such as drawing a picture, writing new code for computer software, or participating in interpretative dance.

Creativity has been shown to decrease stress through focus and concentration. Although this may seem contradictory to the idea of relaxation, creativity can put a person in a "flow state", where all other stressors disappear, and a person can focus solely on their craft. The flow state has been shown to be beneficial by changing our brainwaves, quieting our prefrontal cortex (the area of the brain responsible for self-criticism), and releasing endorphins (Brenner, 2019).

Although we can try and incorporate more creativity into our jobs, it is also helpful to maintain separate creative outlets unrelated to our work.

Social Rest

Social rest may look different depending on your personality type. Although personality typing is not an exact science, it can help us decide where we fall on the spectrum of personality traits, which in turn can be helpful for self-reflection and discovery.

The theories of introversion and extroversion are commonly addressed in many personality tests. Examples of these include the Myers-Briggs Type Indicator (MBTI), Enneagram, and The Holland Codes or the Holland Occupational Themes (RIASEC). The type of rest you enjoy may be a good indicator of whether you are an introvert or extrovert. After interacting with others for many hours, do you find yourself wanting to be alone to decompress? Or would you rather wind down while surrounded by others? Do you find that you feel tired or drained after large social gatherings, or do you feel refreshed and energized by them? These types of questions can help you determine whether you lean more towards the introvert side of the spectrum (alone time replenishes you) or the extrovert end of the spectrum (being around lots of people energizes you). By understanding which way you lean, you can figure out what rest is best for you. Additionally, our moods can change from day to day, affecting how we feel about being around others. Ultimately, self-awareness can help you decide what "social rest" looks like for you.

The type of people we enjoy being around during rest is also essential to consider. While some friends may replenish us, others may be exhausting to hang out with for a more extended period. Take this example:

Samantha is a graduate student who goes to class and works full time. At the end of a long day, she often likes to go home and be alone or spend low-key time with her partner and cat. One evening, as she is leaving class, a classmate she doesn't know well, Emily, approaches her and asks to go to the nearby bar for a quick drink. Samantha is hesitant but ultimately agrees as her partner has recently been telling her to "branch out" more.

Once they arrive at the bar, Emily immediately begins complaining about their professor and the workload he has assigned them. She talks endlessly, so much so that Samantha can barely get a word in edgewise. Samantha finds herself becoming more and more tired as the conversation goes on, as if her life force is being drained from her. Finally, she finishes her drink and leaves Emily with the classic "I need to go feed the cat" excuse.

Samantha tried to branch out with a new friend in this interaction but found herself feeling uncomfortable and exhausted. This feeling could be due to the friend's demeanor, Samantha's long and socially-leaden day, or Samantha's inherent preference for introversion. All of these factors can contribute to our social limits. If Samantha had spent the day lounging alone in her apartment, she might have had a better time with Emily because her limit had not yet been reached. Therefore, when considering what rest looks like for each of us individually, it's essential to view all of these factors to find harmony and balance.

Rest in the Workplace

Psychologically, rest is a mental state free from anything that disrupts peace and serenity (Nurit & Michal 2003). Therefore, workplaces that support regular breaks can decrease accidents, improve worker performance and promote well-being.

One stressor related to the workplace involves the concept of "open loops" or tasks that are never completed, taking up space in our brains. This phenomenon is called the "Zeigarnik Effect". "The Zeigarnik Effect occurs when our attention is negatively affected by incomplete tasks. These incomplete tasks then consume a significant amount of mental energy and resources, creating a series of 'Open Loops' in our minds. In order to assist in helping our brains detach and rest from work, it can be helpful to address and prioritize our tasks, write them down (rather than relying on memory) and avoid opening new loops until we have addressed the already existing loops (Egan, 2019).

One type of journaling that can be particularly helpful in addressing Open Loops is called Bullet Journaling, a specific strategy for addressing tasks in a detailed manner. Bullet journaling may appeal to people that thrive in structured environments and love being organized. An excellent TedTalk on Bullet Journaling can be found in an article written by Reissman (2019), called "How to declutter your mind".

Rest vs. Leisure Activities

Robert is a 27-year old app developer in Silicon Valley. His job is demanding but rewarding, as he loves using his coding skills to create solutions for others. Robert has an educational background in computer science and is well-aware of the detrimental effect too little rest can have. Therefore, he makes a point of going for walks every day to de-stress and get away from his computer.

While on his walks, Robert likes to take photos and post them on Instagram. This social media interaction often leads to a scrolling session to check up on his friends. Often the Instagram session lasts a little longer than intended, and some times he finds himself scrolling throughout the duration of his walk. Although

Robert's walks are an excellent example of leisure activity, he is not benefiting from proper mental rest due to his phone use.

It's essential to distinguish between proper rest and "leisure activities". True rest allows certain parts of the brain to activate and help us stop processing information. One of these brain regions is known as the "default mode network", or DMN. The DMN is important because it helps us focus inward and reconnect with things like our memories, ethics, and creativity. Allowing our DMN to flourish helps us replenish in a way that can be very beneficial.

To activate the DMN, you will need to truly let your mind wander. This idea can seem challenging for many people with high-stress jobs or very active minds. But, remember when you were a child, sitting in the backseat of your parent's car, staring out the window? The action of staring out the window might be the true definition of allowing your mind to wander. Getting back to that feeling can be difficult, but the effects can be life-changing (Cleveland Clinic, 2020).

In contrast, "leisure activities" can also be beneficial. Leisure activities, while still important, are a different type of rest and can include things like reading a book, chatting with a friend, or doing a puzzle. While these activities are refreshing, they are not considered proper mental rest because the brain is still processing information. It should also be noted that being on your phone, scrolling through Instagram, or watching TV is also NOT considered rest because your brain is still processing information.

Now that we've defined different types of rest, we can move on to discovering the benefits of rest. How do humans function at their best when they have enough rest? What types of rest are most beneficial? Where did the American ideas of work and rest originate? All of these questions will be addressed in Chapter 2.

Chapter Two

Why is rest important?

This chapter will cover the positive effects of rest by detailing how humans can function at their best through regular rest. Many studies have shown the impact of rest on cognition, and research suggests that frequent cognitive breaks are needed to sustain focus and performance on mental tasks (Finkbeiner et al., 2016).

Theories of Rest in Occupational Therapy

One of the only health professions that includes rest as a theoretical foundation is Occupational Therapy. OTs assist people in doing everyday activities, and work with various age groups across multiple settings. In addition, occupational Therapists are holistic practitioners, which means they incorporate all aspects of a person's health and the environment when considering patients' needs.

Theoretically, OT is comprised of four categories that contribute to wellness: work, play, sleep, and rest. By balancing these four ideas, healthy life can be achieved. Qualitative research done in this area has led to a greater understanding of what "rest" can mean for different people. The responses truly underline that rest looks different for each person. While some people reported they rested best at home, others said they could only rest while on a trip. Some thought of rest as alone time, while others wanted to be amongst friends. This research is significant as it underscores the importance of integrating regular rest into our everyday lives. Hopefully, as this branch of healthcare becomes more popular, physicians will promote rest as an essential way of maintaining long-term health (Nurit & Avrech Bar, 2003).

What defines a physically rested person?

What happens to our bodies when we get enough rest? Some clues can be taken from athletes. When we rest our bodies, our muscles have time to repair themselves, and glycogen (our body's store of carbohydrates) and fluid levels can replenish. One way to promote physical rest is proactive recovery interventions, including flotation tanks, massages, and saunas. Active rest can also accelerate the recovery process through low-stress exercises such as walking, yoga, or stretching to increase blood flow through the muscles (Kentta & Hassmen, 1998).

We can also better understand the importance of physical rest by taking a cue from high-performance athletes. "Extremely talented people in different disciplines rarely practice more than 4 hours a day on average; subsequent rest and sleep allow the individuals to restore their equilibrium" (Jabr, 2013, para 18).

What defines a mentally rested person?

Mentally rested people purposefully take time out of their day to allow breaks for their brains. It may seem counterintuitive, "purposeful resting", but some people genuinely struggle to sit and let their minds wander. As discussed in Chapter 1, this type of mind-wandering is helpful to activate the "DMN" or Default Mode Network part of our brain.

When we allow the DMN to take over, our brain can access our subconscious. This process is crucial because we connect experiences, thoughts, and actions in ways we might not otherwise do. For example, through this process, we might think about interactions we had during the day with other people, allowing us to form and instill an internal code of ethics or "moral performance review" of sorts. After doing this for some time, people are able to subconsciously solidify their morals and values and better understand how they treat others and how they'd like to improve. Essentially, this type of thinking (or non-thinking) allows us to affirm our identities and decide who we want to become.

The DMN also helps us learn. Our brains can address and solve problems elusive to us during regular mental effort. Studies have shown that engaging in routine activities that don't require much mental effort (such as brushing our teeth) allows us to make better decisions as solutions emerge from our subconscious. This decision-making may be happening due to the brain consolidating information and data, rehearsing recently learned skills, and integrating them into brain tissues. Some studies have also shown that during rest, our brains can strengthen connections between circuits, which can improve memory and attention (Jabr, 2013).

Why is Rest So Difficult for Americans? The History of Rest and Work in America

By understanding the history of work in America, we can better understand why Americans are so uneasy about rest. From the beginning, the importance of work has been drilled into us, alongside a wariness of irresponsible leisure.

In the seventeenth century, America's colonization and settlement by the Puritans brought Victorian ideals of religion and reverence overseas. Puritans viewed hard labor as "a privilege, a glory, and a delight" and often tied work to salvation from God. As it is sometimes called, the "Protestant work ethic" emphasized physically and mentally taxing work for long hours, with a strong disdain for leisure. Some leisure activities were specifically condemned, and colonists caught participating in idleness, dancing, or playing cards were fined or publicly whipped (Hutson, 2012).

After initial colonization, religious motivations for work were replaced with patriotic motives. Rather than working for the glory of God, Americans worked to uphold honor and justice for their country. This attitude was popularized by Benjamin Franklin, who underscored the importance of morals and ethics in the American mindset. Franklin wrote many books on the subject during his lifetime in the eighteenth century. He espoused ideas such as "frugality, industry, justice, chastity, humility, resolution, and order", further cementing the idea of what it meant to be a good person and true American. As a major political figure, Franklin's words had widespread implications, turning personal ethics into a national imperative. Regarding rest and leisure, this is what Benjamin Franklin had to say: "Leisure is the time for doing something useful. This leisure the diligent person will obtain, the lazy one never" (Lasch, 1979).

The Industrial Revolution began in the late eighteenth century and further altered America's motivation for work. As markets became more competitive, so then did workers. The strive for economic success soon overshadowed ethics as factories grew rapidly and people flocked to cities in search of prosperity. Hours became longer, the pace in workplaces became increasingly punishing, and leisure became a luxury unavailable to many. During this industrial boom, Americans found themselves driven to succeed and gave rest and leisure little to no thought (Ciulla, 2000).

Alongside this push for economic success was a desire for Americans to feel as if they were in control of their own destinies. The phrase "rags to riches", introduced by a famous author at the time, promoted the idea that hard work and individualism would lead to success. The premise of "pulling yourself up by your bootstraps" was rampant and instilled in Americans the idea that anything was possible if only they worked hard enough. This mentality placed a heavy burden on people, as their career success was attributed strictly to how hard they worked, ignoring outside influences. This mentality was the first inkling of a message that would take hold and persist throughout American history. Personal identity should hinge on career successes and failures (Packer-Kinlaw, 2013).

This turn towards self-improvement continued throughout the nineteenth century, as did the push towards amassing personal wealth. Prominent figures such as PT Barnum wrote about "The Art of Money-Getting", and excessive wealth became a more common goal for many workers. People were told they could achieve their dreams through self-enrichment, discipline, and self-denial. Sociability and leisure were condemned as they might cause people to miss out on business opportunities (Lasch, 1979).

The twentieth century saw highs and lows for workers. While World Wars I and II brought economic prosperity and increased job opportunities, the Great Depression brought historic lows and unemployment. Amid the Great Depression, government officials and civic leaders worried that the jobless would use their downtime unwisely. This worry led to the creation of structured and organized activities, including the national parks system. In addition, many of the intellectual elites of the Northeast created museums and art galleries in the hope that people would use their time in a responsible way. However, leisure was still viewed as a possible threat to the morals and values of America (McLean & Hurd, 2019).

The 1950s continued America's morality-focused traditions in the workplace with a culture of hierarchy, rule-following, family values, and sacrifice. People also continued working later into their lives, blurring the lines of retirement and relaxation. The 1960s saw an increase in unions within the public sector. This increase led to higher wages, increased job security, and improved living standards for Americans. Unfortunately, this upswing was short-lived. Many labor unions lost their steam in the 1970s when industrial, and manual labor job opportunities waned and were replaced with corporate and private sector jobs. Today, only about 12% of Americans are protected by unions, thus limiting employees' opportunities for self-advocacy and access to benefits (Kuttner, 1992).

In the 1980s and 1990s, the introduction of the internet changed the workplace dramatically, blurring the lines between work and home. Additionally, people were expected to have higher skills for the competitive market, and many jobs required more education. As a result, the mantra of "get a college education so you can get a good job" became commonplace as competition grew more and more fierce within the technology sector (Miller, 2019).

This mantra is still present today, but unfortunately, it holds less true than it used to. Today's workers are overeducated, overworked, and underpaid. For example, "Americans work 137 more hours per year than Japanese workers, 260 more hours per year than British workers, and 499 more hours per year than French workers" (Miller, 2020, para 2).

For most of our history, American values have reflected the importance of work and suspicion of leisure. Americans tie their lives to their jobs, both mentally and physically, as their successes or failures are attributed to their own personal identities. Childcare, medical coverage, and retirement accounts have chained Americans to their jobs to such an extent that they dare not immerse themselves in too much leisure or time off.

The ideas of leisure and rest in America are further eroded in today's Digital Age. Many young workers have found themselves ensconced in "Hustle Culture", and the promotion of "performative workaholism". This trend is particularly true with the rise of social media and technology from the 1990s to today.

Though this example discusses American work habits, many other countries suffer from a culture of overwork. One example is the Japanese idea of "karoshi" which translates to "overwork death". We will discuss the negative implications of too much work and lack of leisure in different countries more fully in Chapter 3.

What defines well-rested workers?

So, how can we distance ourselves from our historical workplace impediments and rigidities? In order to be happier than our predecessors, we need to become purposeful with our time spent at work and our time spent away from work. Utilizing breaks throughout the day is vital.

According to Weir (2019), even "microbreaks" of a few minutes can positively affect people. A study in Korea had telemarketers take relaxation breaks such as stretching or daydreaming, social breaks like chatting with coworkers, and cognitive breaks such as reading the news or watching a video. The results showed that even tiny breaks of just a few minutes lead to increased positive affect at work (i.e., better attitudes). It's also good to note that snack breaks did not have the same effect on positivity! Unfortunately, turning to food for happiness is not an effective way to relax. This study illustrates that even tiny instances of rest can influence our happiness and well-being. Especially in the workplace, it can be beneficial to implement microbreaks.

What should you be doing during your work breaks? This question is essential to consider and is different for each individual. Research shows that people who take breaks to do something they enjoy report fewer health symptoms, like headaches, eye strain, and lower back pain. Additionally, the same people reported higher job satisfaction and lower rates of burnout. The importance here is to decide what makes you happy and participate in that activity during your break. We will go into further detail about hobbies in Chapter 6.

To maximize your rest, you may want to take your breaks in the morning. Because mental resources aren't as drained early in the day, it's easier for people to return to their pre-work levels of happiness and relaxation.

Another critical thing to consider is the effect of taking work home with you. It is essential to detach from work once you leave to get the actual benefits of rest during your time off. In addition, people who experience more psychological detachment from their jobs in their off-hours are more likely to report higher life satisfaction.

Vacations

When thinking about overall physical and mental rest, many of us consider the idea of vacations from work. Many studies have confirmed that vacations are genuinely beneficial to the mind and body through good sleep, less stress, new experiences, and more mind wandering. In addition, workers who take vacations are reported to feel happier, have higher life satisfaction, and be more energetic. Countries with the happiest workers usually have labor laws mandating paid vacation leave. Norway, for example, requires four weeks of vacation time at a minimum, but most companies offer five weeks as the standard (NHO, n.d.).

Unfortunately, the benefits of vacations have been shown to only last for two to four weeks. This data truly helps underscore the importance of taking consistent shorter breaks, as most of us cannot take lengthy vacations every four weeks (Fritz & Sonnentag, 2006).

It is also essential to Maximize specific experiences while on vacation. Scientists have deemed some experiences as "resource-providing" because they help rebuild mental resources that may have been previously drained. In one study, resource-providing experiences included positive work reflection, relaxing activities, and learning something new. It's interesting that learning a new skill while on vacation can contribute positively to our health and wellness. This could be due to the fact that we are removed from work pressures and can learn in an environment without repercussions for failure. So, when planning your ideal vacation, it may be pertinent to think about the types of experiences you want to have. A well-rested vacation could involve some of the "resource-providing" experiences above to maximize rest and recovery processes.

Happiest countries

Every year, researchers compile a "World Happiness Report", which includes rankings based on statistics of the happiest countries. Consistently, Nordic countries rate as the countries with the highest levels of measurable happiness. Much of this can be related to federal policies, such as universal healthcare, free education, and low crime rates. However, Nordic countries also differ from the US in their work-life habits, particularly regarding their emphasis on rest.

In Denmark, full-time employees are given five weeks of vacation regardless of their job sector or title. More importantly, people in Denmark use all of their vacation hours, whereas more than 55% of Americans do not use all of their paid time off. The Danish government also allows for "stress leave", a type of paid disability leave available for people who find themselves in bad work situations that affect their mental health.

So, how can we learn from the Nordic countries? Many of us do not have the means to uproot our lives and head to Denmark. In lieu of that, we should start by using all of our vacation days. This action may feel uncomfortable for many of us, especially Americans, who may view taking time off as a weakness. However, this time is available to be taken. In order to get the rest we need for happiness and health, priorities must be shifted (Stieg, 2020).

Prioritizing rest in the digital age

The negative effects of too much technology are well-documented and will be further covered in the next chapter. First, however, it's also important to consider how the digital age has created opportunities to help us rest in ways that may not have been available before. "Rest-related" technology can be separated into a few categories:

Meditation and Breathing Apps

There are many guided meditation apps that can be helpful for people who feel overwhelmed and busy with their lives. These apps can be set to remind you to breathe, with a notification on your phone (which most of us have on us at all times). These notifications can serve as a helpful reminder throughout the day and keep us on track. There are also meditation apps with a teacher or yogi for guided meditation.

Mental Health Apps

Counselors are more readily available than ever before. Through telehealth, people can connect with a counselor almost immediately when need be. This availability is a massive benefit to busy people who cannot take time off to go to a doctor's office in the middle of their day. Instead, you can find a quiet space in your home, car, or other location to discuss issues with a trained professional.

For some people, the idea of opening up to a stranger may seem too scary and may even provoke more anxiety! Alternative mental health apps allow people to complete activities and learn how to improve their well-being on their own. Many of these apps are based on psychological theories, such as Cognitive Behavioral Therapy, which can help people build skills like gratitude, set goals and challenges, and become more mindful.

Sleep Aids

Sleep aid apps have been created to help us understand the quality and quantity of our sleep. These apps often work by placing your phone on your bedside table or under your pillow. Throughout the night, the app records your movement and breathing to analyze the amount of sleep time spent in REM. These apps can help you understand the quality of your sleep. Other types of sleep-aid apps include those that can stream relaxing nature sounds or white noise. These apps can be particularly beneficial for those who live in noisy cities or crowded apartment complexes.

Wearables

Wearables are exactly what they sound like: technology you wear, including fitness trackers and smartwatches. These devices can give us more insight into our daily activity level, heart rate, blood pressure, and many other metrics.

Organizers

The abundance of organizer apps truly highlights how busy we are as a society. By getting more organized, we can reap the rewards of a decluttered mind, which in turn allows our brains to rest.

Social Apps

Although social media has its downside (again, see next chapter), there is something to be said for the increased connectedness we can now have with our friends and loved ones. Social networks allow us to stay close to those we love when used responsibly and mindfully.

A note on children and technology

Many children grow up surrounded by technology. Although many studies show the unfortunate side effects of this phenomenon, there is still hope. One positive study analyzed children at camp who were away from screens for five days with abundant in-person interaction. At the end of their experience, the children improved significantly in reading the facial emotions of their peers. This skill is invaluable for children's development. It allows them to understand nonverbal emotion and communication with others, affecting how they interact with peers and build relationships. This study is hopeful and shows the importance of screen breaks for children (Uhls et al., 2014).

This chapter taught us the benefits of rest mentally and physically. First, we covered the history of rest and work in America to better understand some of the uneasiness we may have about taking "too much" rest. After looking at how humans can function as their best possible selves, we will now move on to Chapter 3 to discuss the detriments of too little rest.

Chapter Three

What happens if we don't get enough rest?

Now that we've discussed the benefits of rest let's take a look at the consequences of not getting enough rest. Many aspects of our lives can be affected by a lack of rest, including psychological distress, physical injury, and declining job performance. We'll also review different cultural attitudes surrounding the role of rest in our lives and cover the impacts of overwork in various professions.

Mental Consequences

Vigilance and Attention

The "vigilance decrement" is a phenomenon that describes our declining performance in attention the longer we focus on a task. This theory was discovered during WWII when air force radar operators monitored radar screens for enemy submarine activity.

The longer they were on watch, the more mistakes they made (Helton & Russell, 2011).

There are two theories of vigilance decrement currently being debated by scientists: the mindlessness theory and the resource theory. The mindlessness theory posits that monotony in the tasks causes the person to become bored, which leads them to disengage and become preoccupied with their own thoughts. Alternatively, the resource theory focuses more on the information processing systems in our brains and suggests that constant demand depletes these resources and decreases our ability to be vigilant.

Although both theories have merit, the literature suggests that resource theory may be more accurate. For example, in studies of vigilance tasks, participants have reported feeling stressed out and mentally tired at the end of their sessions. These sessions were conducted for minutes, whereas the typical worker is at their job from 6-10 hours per day. This information is helpful for those who may work in highly repetitive jobs that require sustained mental effort, as it underscores the importance of regular breaks throughout the day.

Stress in Relationships

Amanda is a police officer who works the overnight shift three times a week. Her husband Bob works from home as an IT professional. When Amanda has a difficult shift, she likes to come home and talk to Bob about her rough night. Lately, crime has been increasing in her district, and she is facing frequent rough nights. As a result, she finds herself talking to Bob at length almost every day about her struggles.

Bob's job has little to no stress, and he likes it that way. As a champion of work-life balance, Bob finds it easy to disconnect at the end of the day and pursue his hobbies. However, lately, he's beginning to feel dissatisfied with his marriage, unsure why. Assessing the different areas of his life, the only true source of stress he can find is his wife's job, but he's not sure how that could be affecting him. Bob begins to feel increasingly worried about the fate of his marriage if things continue on their current path. He decides to talk to Amanda about how her job affects him and possible solutions.

Chronic stress has been shown to impact romantic relationships negatively. Even daily hassles can lead to tension between partners. When one partner experiences stress from daily hassles, this causes more stress between partners and thus can lead to lower relationship satisfaction. Women's stressors (from within or outside the relationship) tend to have a more substantial effect on the risk for couple dissatisfaction. This difference could be because women tend to communicate more explicitly and openly about their stress than men. Gender differences can also be seen in the level of support provided to the other partner. On stressful days, women still tend to offer more support, whereas men's support also comes with an increase in negative behavior, such as criticizing, blaming, or providing inconsiderate advice (Falconier et al., 2015).

The negative effects stress has on us impact ourselves and our loved ones. In particular, the impact on our partners underscores the importance of minimizing stress through self-care and rest.

Physical Consequences

According to the American Psychological Association (2018), continuous stress affects all parts of our bodies:

Musculoskeletal System

Constant stress affects the musculoskeletal system and results in muscle tension, which is the body's way of protecting itself against injury and pain. Muscle tension can show up in different body parts, including the shoulders and back, and may manifest as tension headaches. Migraine headaches are debilitating to many people and also associated with chronic stress.

Respiratory System

The respiratory system supplies oxygen to the body and removes carbon dioxide waste. Stress can present as shortness of breath and rapid breathing and can also exacerbate pre-existing respiratory problems like chronic obstructive pulmonary disease, emphysema, and chronic bronchitis. In addition, for those of us who already suffer from physical illnesses like asthma or mental illnesses like panic disorder, extensive stress can cause attacks.

Cardiovascular System

Acute stress, or situationally-based stress, is momentary and short-term. It can happen in response to a sudden catalyst, such as a bee landing on you or slamming on your brakes to avoid an accident. This type of stress increases your heart rate and intensifies your heart muscle contractions. Additionally, blood vessels that direct blood to your heart dilate, or open, which increases the amount of blood being pumped to specific body parts. This reaction is known as a "fight or flight response" and causes an elevation in blood pressure.

Long-term stress can contribute to elevated blood pressure for a prolonged period, increasing the risk of hypertension, heart attack, or stroke. These increased risks are thought to be related to inflammation within the circulatory system and increased cholesterol levels in response to chronic stress.

It's important to note that stress affects women's cardiovascular systems differently depending on age. For example, premenopausal women respond better to stress, which protects them from heart disease. In contrast, postmenopausal women lose this level of protection as their estrogen levels drop, making them more susceptible to heart disease.

Endocrine System

When people are put into stressful situations, a part of their brain called the hypothalamic-pituitary-adrenal (HPA) axis goes into overdrive. The HPA produces steroid hormones called glucocorticoids, including cortisol (the "stress hormone").

Although cortisol is released in our body regularly throughout the day to help us function correctly, stressful situations cause our HPAs to produce an excess of cortisol to provide energy so we can respond to extreme situations. This increased production is valuable and necessary when we are in extreme situations. Still, chronic stress can confuse our bodies into thinking they are in extreme situations continuously, leading to an excess of cortisol in our bodies.

The HPA also communicates with our immune system to reduce inflammation. Chronic stress impairs communication between the HPA and the immune system, lowering our immune response through decreased regulation. This impaired communication has been connected to the development of future conditions, including chronic fatigue, diabetes, obesity, immune disorders, and depression.

Gastrointestinal System

The gut has hundreds of millions of neurons in continuous communication with the brain. Chronic stress affects this communication, triggering pain, bloating, and discomfort. The gut is also inhabited by bacteria that affect gut and brain health and can impact thinking and emotions. While under stress, our gut bacteria changes, which can influence our moods.

Chronic stress can cause us to eat more or less than usual and affect the types of foods we crave. Additionally, coping mechanisms such as tobacco or alcohol can lead to heartburn or acid reflux. Stress can also negatively affect our swallowing reflex, which leads to more air being swallowed. This change, in turn, increases burping, gas, and bloating.

Stress can cause pain, bloating, nausea and discomfort more easily and can even result in vomiting if the stress is severe enough. However, it is a myth that stress causes an increase in acid production and leads to ulcers. Ulcers are actually caused by bacterial infections.

Also affected are our bowels and digestion processes. Food may move more quickly or slowly through our intestines, resulting in constipation or diarrhea. Our intestines may also have a more challenging time absorbing nutrients from food, leading to us feeling poorly because our bodies are not receiving what they need to function well.

Nervous System

The nervous system is made up of several divisions: the brain and spinal cord are included in the central division, and the autonomic and somatic nervous systems fall under the peripheral division.

Here, we will focus on the autonomic nervous system, which plays a vital role in modulating stress reactions.

Autonomic Nervous System

The Autonomic Nervous System is further divided into the Sympathetic Nervous System (SNS) and the Parasympathetic Nervous System (PNS). These two systems balance each other, as the SNS helps the body respond to the emergency, and the PNS assists in returning the body to a normal state.

When we are under stress, the SNS creates a fight or flight response and shifts its energy resources to address the perceived enemy. The fight or flight response happens when the SNS releases hormones such as adrenaline and cortisol. These hormones cause the heart to beat quicker, the breathing rate to increase, blood vessels to dilate, and the digestive process to change to increase glucose (sugar energy) levels in the bloodstream.

When the crisis passes, the PNS assists the body to get back to its pre-emergency state. However, when we face chronic stress, the PNS can become overactive, resulting in bronchoconstriction (asthma attacks) or compromised blood circulation.

Chronic stress negatively affects the autonomic nervous system as it causes wear and tears on the body. In addition, the continuous activation of these systems has a strong effect on the immune system, which over time exhausts our bodies and leads to poorer functioning in many bodily functions.

Reproductive Systems

Women

Women are affected by chronic stress in many different ways. For example, premenopausal women may miss their periods, have irregular menstrual cycles, or suffer more painful periods. Chronic stress can also affect women's sex drives, which can lead to relationship and self-esteem issues.

Pregnancy is also significantly impacted by chronic stress. Women under constant stress can have a much harder time conceiving, and they are more susceptible to postpartum issues such as depression and anxiety. Maternal stress can also lead to fetal and childhood development problems and disrupt mother-baby bonding after delivery.

Men

The nervous system influences the male reproductive system. The PNS causes relaxation, and the SNS causes arousal. Chronic stress can affect these systems, leading to lower testosterone production, a decline in sex drive, erectile dysfunction, or impotence.

Ongoing stress can also affect sperm production, sperm motility, and sperm size and shape. Research has shown that even just two stressful life events within a year can affect sperm negatively. These effects can contribute to relationship issues and further promote a stress cycle for couples trying to conceive (Cohen et al., 2007).

Burnout

According to Michel (2016), the term "burnout" was coined in 1974 to describe volunteers working at a free clinic in New York City. The mental health workers in a clinic were struggling with emotional depletion, loss of motivation, and increased cynicism. Today, burnout is so prevalent that mainstream medicine has recognized it. There is a large degree of overlap between this condition and depression, including fatigue, loss of passion, and intensifying negativity.

Burnout relates to stress levels often created by job duties overpowering a person's ability to cope with stress. The careers reporting the most burnout include the caregiving careers, such as nurses, doctors, social workers, and teachers (sometimes referred to as "compassion fatigue", particularly in the mental health field). Research shows that the top six components contributing to burnout are: workload, control, reward, community, fairness, and values. Burnout happens when one or more of these areas is consistently mismatched between a person and their job.

Several interesting studies have shown the correlation between burnout and brain functioning. For example, one study measured the connections between the amygdala (a structure that regulates emotional reactions) and the anterior cingulate cortex (ACC), which is an area of the brain linked to emotional distress. The more stressed an individual reported feeling, the weaker the connectivity between these brain regions. This discovery is just one example of how continuous stress in our workplaces can contribute to structural changes in our brains and increased negativity and hopelessness.

Luckily, the symptoms of burnout and chronic stress can be reversed. For example, a study in the US examined stressed students studying for the US medical licensing exam and found that their abilities in attention switching were impaired. These students were again examined four weeks after completing their exams and after they had time to rest. This time, the group returned to their normal attention patterns.

Although the symptoms of burnout can be scary, it's hopeful that they can be reversed. Evaluating our jobs and stress levels is essential, and regular rest from these stressors is imperative to promote healthy mental functioning.

Job-Related Problems

A lack of rest can affect different occupations in different ways. Let's take a look at how surgeons, judges, and pilots can all be affected by chronic stress:

Surgeons:

Although surgeons often cite stress as a key factor in their training and practice, too much stress can lead to errors. Too much stress in surgery can result in physical symptoms, such as loss of dexterity, clumsiness, and physical tension. Emotionally, surgeons experience anxiety, anger, frustration, and irritability. Cognitively, surgeons have reported indecisiveness and an inability to think clearly. Behaviorally, surgeons inadvertently may find themselves becoming more short-tempered with their support staff as their communication skills break down (Wetzel et al., 2006).

Physical and mental rest are often used as coping strategies in the operating room. For example, surgeons may "stand back mentally" to regain self-control. During complex procedures, surgeons may also take a break from an intricate part of the surgery and move on to a different concern, planning to return later to the tricky part. Physically, surgeons employ deep breathing, temporary distancing from the patient, and positive self-talk. Additionally, it has been shown that "microbreaks" for long surgeries are particularly beneficial for surgeons' physical wellness. These breaks can include posture correction and certain types of stretching that allow surgeons to stay sterile (Coleman Wood et al., 2018).

Flight crews:

Both cabin crews and pilots are subject to fatigue-related issues in their jobs. For example, problems reported from working international flights include increased weight gain, lowered immune function, and inability to function at home upon immediate return. Additionally, crew members have reported that increased irritability, decreased alertness, and uncontrollable bouts of falling asleep have affected performance.

Insufficient rest for the crew was the major contributor to the above issues. Work-life balance is difficult for the crew to maintain, as they cannot balance the time commitments required for this type of work with family obligations and proper sleep. Some recommendations for improving rest for flight crews include splitting breaks between employees, improving rest facilities, and changing roster schedules to optimize time for rest (Van Den Berg et al., 2019).

Judges:

Judges have demanding jobs that require intense, consistent attention and decisiveness. Research shows that making repeated decisions can deplete an individual's executive functioning and cognitive resources (see "vigilance decrement" above for more information). Making repeated rulings may also increase the likelihood of taking shortcuts, such as simplifying decisions or accepting the status quo to reduce mental burdens.

Judges who take regular breaks are more likely to make favorable rulings. Favorable rulings are more likely when judges are well-rested, and their cognitive resources are full at the beginning of the day. Fair decisions also are more likely to happen after a food break (although it is undetermined whether the break, the food, or both is the main factor here) (Danziger et al., 2011).

Cultural differences when it comes to rest:

Our culture can dictate our attitudes towards rest in the workplace. In the last chapter, we discussed American work culture and the negative attitudes many Americans hold when it comes to rest. Here, we'll explore other cultures and their views on rest (DiOrio, 2019):

Japan

Overwork in Japan is such a common occurrence that the Japanese have coined a term for death from overwork: karoshi. The first instance of karoshi occurred in 1969 when a male worker in a shipping department of Japan's largest newspaper company died due to a stroke. The Ministry of Labor found that his death was caused by night shift work and increased workload despite his ill health. Since then, Japan has documented many more cases of karoshi, with the most common causes of death being heart attack and stroke.

Workplaces are beginning to encourage mid-day breaks and sleep, called hirune in Japanese, to combat this frightening epidemic.

Some companies have even created facilities for napping or relaxing that offer a quiet environment and a collection of reclining chairs (Shibata, 2019).

France

France's government promotes work-life balance through federal legislation. For example, laws in France require a maximum 35-hour workweek and a minimum of five weeks of vacation. The government also passed a new policy that gives employees the right to disconnect from work-related email and other communications when they are not physically present in the office. France also has a strong union presence, allowing employee protection and advocacy (DiOrio, 2019).

South Korea

South Korea also has a term for "death by overwork": gwarosa. South Koreans work more hours every week than almost any other country. Recently, as the government has become more concerned about its citizens, a new law was put in place for office workers to lower their workweek from 68 hours per week to 40 hours per week. Although this is a step in the right direction, the law only applies to companies with over 300 employees (DiOrio, 2019).

Spain

Spain, known for its "siestas" or mid-day naps, is taking steps to change this practice. Although Spaniards work long hours, two to three of those hours are usually spent at lunch. Unfortunately, this practice has led to lower productivity in Spain and slower economic growth.

Cyberclick has effectively addressed this issue by having no set working schedule for its employees. As long as employees meet their goals, they can work as many hours per week as they want and still get paid their predetermined salary. Teams can also decide how much holiday they want to take each year and can telework as much as they like (Park, 2019).

Americans are often victims of "hustle culture", which is the mentality that we must continue our work until it's done, sacrificing sleep, breaks, and well-being. This mentality causes guilt when we take breaks and pervasive stress. Looking at some of the patterns from other cultures, government mandates regarding maximum hours worked and mandatory vacation are essential factors in employee happiness. Additionally, an office culture that allows flexibility and promotes trust among employees can lead to happier workers (Headversity, n.d.).

Are we more at risk for lack of rest in the digital age?

Billy is in his mid-30s and works for a fast-paced startup full time. His job is draining, but he feels he's got a good handle on his work-life balance. At lunch with his friend Eric, Billy makes sure to put his phone on vibrate. He places it on the table, face down, so as not to be distracted.

At the end of lunch, Eric looks concerned and asks Billy if his job is getting to be too much for him. Billy is confused and wonders why Eric would think such a thing. He purposely put his phone on vibrate so his lunch with his friend wouldn't be interrupted! Eric pointed out that Billy picked up his phone to check for notifications about 20 times during lunch. He says he felt like

Billy wasn't hearing him during their conversation, which made him feel unimportant.

Billy wasn't even aware that he had checked his phone so many times. He had no idea that the very presence of his phone on the table was causing the conversation to be superficial and unfulfilling for his friend. He plans to invite Eric for a make-up dinner and intends to leave his phone in the car.

While the benefits of technology are numerous, the detriments are also abundant. For example, constantly being around our devices has affected our communication abilities, stress levels, and cognition. Additionally, the increased opportunities for working from home have had positive and negative effects on well-being.

Most of us always have our phones on or near us. Unfortunately, research has shown that the presence of cell phones has negative effects on closeness, connection, and conversation quality (Misra et al., 2014). This research suggests that having your phone in your hand or on the table when conversing with someone else can lead to lower levels of empathy and a diminished quality of conversation (Ward et al., 2017). Additionally, those who constantly check their phones have a higher risk for increased stress levels (American Psychological Association, 2017).

During the COVID-19 pandemic, many companies began offering flexible working arrangements, including the option to work from home. Although many people report positive side effects of working from home, this option may also be promoting "presenteeism", or working even when it might not be the best thing for you (Lufkin, 2019). Many people still bring themselves to the office when they aren't feeling well, and with the ability to work from home, workers may be doing this even more frequently. With available technology at home, employees may be tempted to save their precious sick hours in favor of pushing through the pain (Przybylski & Weinstein, 2012).

The implications of this research are essential to consider when we plan our breaks. If we turn to our devices for rest, this may not be offering the same level of relaxation as technology-free activities. Digital dependence is a real issue, and taking breaks from our phones may improve our relationships and, paradoxically, our social connections. Additionally, work-from-home options may benefit certain people but not necessarily everyone. It's important to consider our abilities to disconnect from work. Are you a person who can draw these boundaries when working from home, or would you feel better about disconnecting if you can physically leave your office?

Now that we have covered what happens when we don't get enough rest in various contexts, let's take a look at the importance of sleep.

Chapter Four

Sleep

Collin is a manager at a prestigious marketing firm. He oversees twelve employees and is responsible for advocating for them. One day at work, the manager of another team, May, chastises a member of Collin's team. Collin discovers this interaction through the grapevine and thinks about how to confront May. The issue is challenging because he needs to be firm but diplomatic. He considers the problem all day and goes to sleep uneasy and anxious.

When he wakes up in the morning, Collin remembers fragments of his dreams, but they disappear quickly. He gets up and makes tea while mentally preparing for his day. As the water is boiling, an idea floats into his mind about handling his work situation. It is a brilliant idea, and he feels confident it will efficiently solve the problem without alienating anyone.

In this example, dreaming may have solved Collin's problem. Let's look into the reasons why we sleep in order to understand the numerous benefits it brings.

Why do we sleep

For decades, scientists have been trying to answer the elusive question: why do we sleep? There are several leading theories, and scientists believe that more than one of them may contribute to the answer (Harvard Medical School, 2007):

Inactivity Theory

This theory, based in evolutionary science, was one of the earliest theories of sleep. It posits that inactivity during the night allows organisms to be safely out of harm's way during a vulnerable time by enabling them to stay still and quiet. Through natural selection, this strategy evolved to become sleep.

Energy Conservation Theory

Natural selection favors organisms that use less energy because they need fewer resources (food) to survive. This theory suggests that sleep is utilized to reduce an organism's energy demands. Metabolism is reduced during sleep due to decreased body temperature and caloric demand. The fewer resources an organism needs, the more likely they are to survive.

Restorative Theories

Restorative theories suggest that sleep serves to restore resources that are lost while we are awake. There is strong empirical support for this theory: animals deprived entirely of sleep lose their immune functions altogether and die within weeks. Additionally, other vital processes in the body, such as muscle growth, protein synthesis, and tissue repair, occur mainly, or exclusively, during sleep.

Cognitively, our brain also seems to need restoration. During the day, our brains produce adenosine. When adenosine builds up, we begin to feel tired. Research suggests that this buildup may promote a "drive to sleep". Our body can clear adenosine buildups during sleep, and we can feel more alert during the waking hours.

Brain Plasticity Theory

This newer theory is based on findings that correlate sleep with changes in the structure and organization of the brain. Infant sleep patterns can support this theory. Infants sleep up to 14 hours per day, which plays a critical role in their brain development. In adults, the effects of sleep can be seen in various tasks, such as learning and memory.

Dreaming

Research suggests that dreaming is essential for our psychological well-being. Dreams can help us take the edge off of traumatic events by allowing us to view them from a distance while asleep. REM sleep is beneficial because it is the only time our brain is entirely free from the anxiety-triggering hormone noradrenaline, so we can mentally experience our difficult experiences from the day without becoming triggered. Dreaming can also enhance our creative problem-solving abilities and help us consolidate memories (Walker, 2017).

Evolution of Sleep Patterns

Why are some people early birds and others night owls? Evolution may be the cause. Anthropologists have posited that because our ancestors lived in groups, it made sense for someone to be on the lookout for predators at all times. Over time, this could have affected our genetics so that our current body clocks are descended from either those night owls or early birds.

Age is also thought to be an essential factor in sleep. The "Grandmother Hypothesis" suggests that it was beneficial for our ancestors to have older people in the group. Older people tend to wake at night, need less sleep, and get up earlier. These habits of older people could have been helpful for our ancestors, as they would have had a lookout when others were usually sleeping (Briggs, 2017).

Consequences of Sleep Deprivation

When we talk about sleep deprivation, it's important to note the recommendations for sleep. Adults should focus on getting 7-8 hours of sound sleep per night. What constitutes sound sleep will be covered later in this chapter. Consistent sleep deprivation can cause various issues and can have far-reaching effects on our lives (Colten & Altevogt, 2006).

Mental and Emotional Issues

Adults with chronic sleep loss may suffer from more significant depressive symptoms, anxiety, and mental distress. In addition to the above symptoms, teenagers who get inadequate sleep are more likely to have behavioral problems, lower self-esteem, and a higher risk for attempted suicide.

A study from Australia analyzed the quality of sleep and the effects of sleep deprivation on a group of people suffering from mental illness. The study concluded that "the prevalence of suboptimal sleep is approximately twice as high among people with a mental health condition in Australia, compared to those without such a condition". Those who already deal with mental health issues may be at a higher risk of poor sleep and the associated detrimental effects.

Physical Issues

People who consistently don't get enough sleep are subject to a wide range of physical ailments. These include obesity, diabetes, cardiovascular disease, high blood pressure, and increased possibility of alcohol use (Metst et al., 2021).

Sleep Debt

People who consistently do not get enough sleep can have what's called "sleep debt". As we know, adults should get at least seven hours of sleep per night. So, if we were only to get 5 hours of sleep one night, this would mean a debt of two hours to make up. In addition, sleep debt is considered cumulative, so even if we go to sleep 30 or 60 minutes later than usual for just a few days, those hours can quickly add up.

We can make up our sleep debt by taking naps of ten to twenty minutes in the early morning or mid-afternoon. However, it is unclear whether sleeping in on the weekends is beneficial for sleep debt. Although we may "catch up", we also disrupt our sleep routine, which is an essential part of sleep hygiene.

Research has shown that sleep debt can take some time to be repaid. For example, we may need four days to recover from one hour of lost sleep. In addition, our body may require up to nine days to eliminate our sleep debt entirely (Newsom & Rehman, 2021).

Sleep Disorders

Sleep disorders can contribute to chronic sleep deprivation. Some of these disorders include (Cleveland Clinic, n.d.):

Sleep Apnea

There are two types of Sleep Apnea, obstructive sleep apnea (OSA) and central sleep apnea (CSA). OSA is more common and is caused by a blockage of the airway in the throat. OSA sufferers are usually loud snorers and may gasp for air while sleeping. Other symptoms include daytime sleepiness, fatigue, and trouble concentrating. In CSA, the brain fails to tell the body to breathe during sleep, which leads to constant awakenings during the night.

Sleep apnea is very harmful, as it lessens the amount of air our bodies can get while asleep. Many people don't even know that they suffer from it. If you are a loud snorer and suffer from any of the symptoms above, you may want to consider having a sleep study to get diagnosed.

Insomnia

Insomnia is a sleep disorder where people have trouble either staying asleep or falling asleep. About 50% of adults experience occasional insomnia, but one in ten have chronic insomnia. Short-term insomnia can be caused by stress, illness, or environmental factors. Long-term insomnia can be caused by underlying conditions, such as depression, chronic stress, or anxiety.

Restless Legs Syndrome

Restless legs syndrome (RLS) causes intense urges to move the legs, often brought on by resting or prolonged periods of sitting. Often, people with RLS feel they need to walk around and shake their legs for relief, which is disruptive during sleep hours.

Narcolepsy

Narcolepsy is a neurological disorder that causes people to experience excessive daytime sleepiness. People with this condition may also fall asleep uncontrollably during the daytime. In addition, some patients may experience sudden muscle weakness or extreme emotional outbursts.

Sleep Walking

Sleepwalking occurs more often in children, but adults with a family history may also be prone to episodes. Sleepwalking often occurs early in the night (shortly after falling asleep) and is unlikely to occur during naps. As a result, people who sleepwalk may do routine activities around their house, engage in unusual behavior, become violent immediately after waking, and not remember the episode in the morning. Night terrors (episodes of extreme fear, screaming, or flailing while asleep) may also occur alongside sleepwalking (Mayo Clinic, n.d.).

Shift Work Disorder

Certain occupations are at a greater risk of sleep loss, particularly occupations that require night shifts. These professions include nurses, truck drivers, and air cabin crews, amongst others. Research has consistently shown that many workers in these fields are subject to shift work disorder, "a circadian rhythm sleep disorder characterized by excessive sleepiness, insomnia, or both as a result of shift work". In addition, those of us who identify as "morning people" may also suffer more from working the night shift due to our specific circadian rhythms (Magnavita & Garabarino, 2017).

Consequences of Too Much Sleep

Too much sleep is also associated with harm. One study from the United Kingdom suggests that too much sleep may be worse than too little sleep. The study analyzed different amounts of sleep, between 4 hours and 10 hours, and found a J-shaped relationship between hours of sleep and risk of death. For example, if 7-8 hours of sleep correlates to a "normal" amount of risk of death, then the risk rises at 6 hours and goes even higher at 4 hours. Comparatively, the risk increases after 8 hours and substantially spikes at 10 hours.

This study is critical because it helps us understand the optimal sleep window of 7-8 hours. Even if we may not want to wake up after 8 hours, sleeping more than that could shorten our lifespans (Kwok et al., 2018).

Sleep Hygiene

Getting good sleep is an essential part of rest and replenishment. Quality sleep can be defined as uninterrupted sleep and results in feeling refreshed and awake in the morning and during the following day. Good sleep is promoted by sleep hygiene, which is akin to regular hygiene in that we need to make an effort to practice these habits consistently.

Sleep hygiene looks different for everyone, but it should include some important aspects such as going to bed and waking up at the same time every day (even on weekends), unplugging from technology at least an hour before bed (blue light can interfere with our sleep quality), and making the bedroom a place where quality sleep can occur. The light in the bedroom should be at a minimum, blue lights should be covered, the room should be kept cool (around 65 degrees Fahrenheit or 18 degrees Celsius), and the space should be quiet.

Other ideas to consider for your nighttime routine include essential oils in a diffuser or scented flameless candles. Although the effects of essential oils have not been well-studied, many people report feelings of calm and contentment. In addition, some light sleepers may enjoy white noise machines or earplugs to promote uninterrupted sleep by blocking out ambient noises like their partner snoring (Walker, 2017).

Do electronic devices and technology affect the quality of our sleep?

Utilizing electronic devices before bed can impact the quality of our sleep. Here, we refer to electronic devices that use blue light, such as cell phones, computers, iPads, and televisions. This collection of devices does not necessarily include eReaders such as the Kindle, as they work differently.

To understand how these devices affect our sleep, we'll first define circadian rhythms. Circadian rhythms are changes in our bodies that follow a 24-hour cycle. These processes influence essential functions in our body, such as hormone release, digestion, and body temperature. Circadian rhythms also control our sleep by producing a hormone called melatonin. Our brains produce melatonin in response to incoming light processed via optic nerves. When there is less light, the brain makes more melatonin, and we get drowsy (National Institute of General Medical Sciences, n.d.).

So how does blue light affect our circadian rhythms? Because light is the most critical environmental signal impacting the circadian clock, it would make sense that utilizing a lighted device before bedtime would affect our sleep quality. One experiment studied the effects of bedtime reading on an iPad instead of a paperback book in dim lighting. The study found that the circadian rhythms of those who utilized the iPad were altered, which resulted in more trouble falling asleep, later sleep times, and reduced alertness in the morning of the following day. The iPad group also had lower levels of measured melatonin and reduced REM sleep (Chang et al., 2014).

This study, and many others, validate the effects of blue light on our sleep. For those of us who browse social media on our phones while in bed at night, it may be helpful to consider its effect on our sleep quality and long-term health. Alternatives to late-night technology use can include paperback books or magazines and devices designed to be utilized in the evening (such as eReaders that do not emit blue light). In addition, screens should be avoided two to three hours before bed, and in the evenings, dim red lights can work well, as red light is less likely to shift our circadian rhythms (Harvard Health Publishing, 2020).

As we've seen in this chapter, good sleep is essential to our physical and mental well-being. Next, we'll look into other ways of promoting health through exercise and sports.

Chapter Five

Exercise

Exercise has long been known to be beneficial to our health. So let's look at the numerous benefits it can provide.

How much exercise do we need?

According to the World Health Organization (WHO, 2020), there are different recommendations for how much exercise we need based on age group:

Infants less than 1 year old

Babies should be physically active through floor-based play or tummy time if they are not yet mobile. Additionally, they should not be restrained for more than 1 hour at a time (highchairs, strollers, etc.).

Children 1-4 years of age

Children at this age should spend at least 180 minutes participating in various physical activities spread throughout the day.

Children and teens 5-17 years of age

This age group should aim to average 60 minutes of moderate to vigorous activity per day, including aerobic activity and strengthening activities.

Adults 18-64 years of age

Adults should aim for 150-300 minutes of moderate-intensity activity or 75-150 minutes of vigorous-intensity activity per week. Two days per week should also include moderate or intense muscle-strengthening activities.

Adults 65+ years of age

Adults in this age group should aim for the same amount of activity as the 18-64 age group. However, adults 65+ should emphasize balance and strength training to enhance functional capacity and minimize the risk of falls.

The WHO also recommends that pregnant and postpartum women participate in at least 150 minutes of moderate-intensity aerobic activity per week. In addition, women in this category should limit the amount of time spent being inactive and replace idle time with physical activity (even light activity).

Benefits of Exercise

The benefits exercise has on our bodies, and mental health is invaluable. Let's take a closer look at some of these.

Brain

The brain benefits from exercise just as much as the body does. For older adults, exercise can lower the risk of developing dementia and Alzheimer's disease, two types of degenerative diseases. Specifically, exercise helps our brains improve memory and thinking skills and can lower the risk for dementia by up to 31%. Research has also been done on adults already suffering from mild cognitive impairment. For example, in one study, which lasted for six months, 160 older people were assigned to follow a specific diet only or follow the diet and exercise. The results showed improved thinking and memory for the group that exercised. In contrast, there was no change in executive functioning (planning, problem-solving, multitasking) for the group that followed the diet alone.

Exercise works to help the brain through various avenues. Improved blood flow to the brain, reduced inflammation, and lowered stress hormones are a few examples of how exercise can alter our brains for the better. Exercise can also physically alter our brain structures by promoting neuroplasticity, which helps our brains adapt as we age.

The idea of "mental exercise" is also intriguing for brain health. Research suggests that mentally stimulating activities, such as learning a new skill or doing a crossword puzzle, can help build our "cognitive reserves". These reserves allow us to be more resilient to adverse brain changes as we age and act as protective measures. In addition, continuously learning new things and engaging in intellectually stimulating environments can help our brains create more connections between different areas of our brains, which allows us to remain more functional the older we get (Cleveland Clinic, 2019).

Body

Our bodies benefit from all types of exercise, from walking to weightlifting. People who do not participate in sufficient exercise increase their risk of mortality by 20 to 30 percent. Regular physical activity improves cardiorespiratory fitness and can reduce the chances of heart diseases, cancer, stroke, and diabetes. Weight training can also help us improve our strength, which helps us be more functional in our everyday lives.

Exercise can also help us maintain a healthy weight, lowering our risk of some diseases, including diabetes. Being active boosts the "good" kind of cholesterol, high-density lipoprotein (HDL), and decreases unhealthy triglycerides in our blood. Exercise can also enhance sexual arousal for women and reduce erectile dysfunction for men.

As discussed in the last chapter, good sleep is essential for our well-being. Exercise promotes better sleep in a number of ways and leads to deeper sleep and the ability to fall asleep faster. However, it is important not to exercise too close to bedtime as this can lead to difficulty falling asleep due to increased energy (WHO, 2020).

Mental Health

Kierstin is a thirty-year-old teacher who works in a challenging school district. Her bosses often pile on more work than is necessary, and they are inflexible with her requests even though she is an excellent practitioner.

Lately, Kierstin has been struggling with feelings of sadness and apathy. She is losing interest in her job and the only thing keeping her going is her connection with her students. One of her coworkers, Amber, has recently started a running club and invites Kierstin to join. Kierstin ran almost every day in college and loved it, so she decided to participate.

After two weeks of running with the group, Kierstin has noticed that her mental health has changed for the better. When she wakes up in the morning, her outlook is more positive, and she no longer dreads the drive to work. She decides to commit to keep running with the group, as her mental health has dramatically improved.

Our mental health can be improved by exercise through a reduction in our sensitivity to stress. Exercise does not necessarily reduce stress, but rather it can increase our tolerance to stress and improve resiliency. There are several theories as to why and how exercise can improve our mental health. Some suggest that mental health improves gradually through feelings of self-mastery and social integration. Others cite antidepressant and anti-anxiety actions in the brain that lead to improved mood (Salmon, 2001).

Longer Life

Exercise can increase our lifespan. Studies have shown that we should take at least 7,000 steps a day to improve our longevity. The correct amount of physical activity can reduce our chances of premature death by up to 70%. However, there seems to be an upper limit to the number of steps that benefit us. When we walk more than 10,000 steps a day, the benefits seem to plateau. When looking at other types of exercise, about 2.5 hours a week roughly translates to 7,000 steps per day, and 4.5 hours a week is equal to about 10,000 steps (Reynolds, 2021).

Why is it so hard for many of us to exercise?

Even though we know about the multitude of benefits of exercise, many of us still struggle to do it. Why is this? One theory of this struggle is based in evolutionary psychology. Our ancestors partly survived because they aimed to avoid unnecessary physical activity, thus decreasing their need for resources. Because hunter-gatherers walked about six miles a day searching for food, they compensated by being as inactive as possible during their downtime. This past could be one possible reason for our modern-day aversion to exercise.

Looking to our ancestors can help us learn ways to get around this aversion. Humans evolved to be endurance runners. With short toes, arched feet, long tendons, and large gluteal muscles, we are uniquely equipped to be excellent runners. Humans are also adapted not to overheat through a multitude of sweat glands. While understanding our physical adaptations may not be sufficient to get us to exercise, thinking about why our ancestors chose to be active is helpful. Humans evolved to exercise when necessary or fun. For example, in almost all human cultures, dancing is a tradition. Relating this to exercise, we can make our exercise fun by working out with friends or choosing exercises that create joy (King, 2020).

How to Build an Exercise Habit

For many of us, building new habits can be challenging. This same challenge also applies to exercise. However, we can utilize behavioral science factors to help us develop better habits (Milkman & Duckworth, 2018). Below are some scientifically backed methods for creating an exercise habit:

1. Build accountability by exercising with other people – Research shows that people are more likely to exercise if they have scheduled a workout with another person. This scheduling is effective because it holds us accountable to someone else, whereas we may not feel as strongly about holding ourselves accountable on our own. People also

enjoy doing the same things as their friends, which can help build the habit even more.

2. Pick a good day to start – Motivation can ebb and flow throughout the year, so picking a day that may already hold significance can help jumpstart a new habit. A new year, a new week or a meaningful day like a birthday can all be good choices.

3. Set a challenging goal that allows for flexibility – The most effective goals are goals that are tough but not impossible. Setting an ambitious goal, but allowing for wiggle room, is a valuable type of goal. An example of this would be a goal of working out daily, with a built-in "free pass" if you miss a day or two during a given week. It's also important not to be too hard on ourselves when we sometimes fall short.

4. Try to reach your goal for at least a month – Research has shown that it takes a month to build a lasting habit. Once we set a goal, it's essential to keep working towards that goal for one month to have the best shot at sticking to it.

5. Use all available resources – We have access to more online resources than ever before in our current digital age. The benefits of online fitness classes and resources include access for all people regardless of their proximity to a gym. These classes are also helpful for parents and busy business people who may not have the time to drive to other locations. Exercise classes can be found for just about every fitness level, and some of them are even free. We can find classes that match our strengths and interests

while not spending any money. Additionally, habit trackers and planning apps can help us stay accountable to ourselves and others.

Exercise Around the World

Attitudes surrounding exercise differ throughout the world. The World Health Organization (WHO) released a report analyzing people's fitness levels in 168 countries from 2001 to 2016. The report found that among rich Western countries, Finland was the fittest. Overall, Uganda was number one globally (Brueck, 2019).

Uganda's fitness levels are due to various factors, one of which is that many Ugandans have physically demanding jobs, which may be less prevalent in wealthier countries. Another factor is that Ugandans can spend a lot of time walking to and from work. This exercise comes in addition to physical exertion at their jobs. Generally, people in lower-income countries automatically integrate more physical activity into their lives out of necessity. It has been postulated that as a country becomes wealthier, its citizens may become unhealthier as they enjoy more luxuries such as accessible transportation, sedentary jobs, and greater access to food (BBC News, 2018).

Within western civilization, Finland leads in fitness. 56% of Finnish adults (30-64 years old) get at least one hour of moderately intense activity per day. This habit is partly due to Finnish attitudes towards wellness, but the country also provides social safety nets that allow citizens to focus on their fitness. For example, Finnish employers spend an average of $220 per year on their employees' fitness, including saunas, gyms, and gym vouchers (Brueck, 2019).

Exercise in different age groups

Jordan is 70 years old and retired. He exercises every day by going for walks around the park with his dog. He also does yoga three times a week and focuses on flexibility. Jordan's friend Ron recently had a bad fall and ended up breaking his hip. Now that Ron is on the mend, he wants to exercise because his doctor recommended it for his recovery. Jordan invites Ron to walk with him every morning, and Ron's doctor thinks this is an excellent idea, especially for someone in his age group. Jordan is happily surprised to learn that his regular exercise habit is actually recommended! He hopes to help his friend begin on his new healthy journey and continue to keep himself fit.

Let's explore what exercise can look like in different age groups.

Elderly

Exercise is essential regardless of age but can be especially beneficial for older people. Because this age group is most susceptible to falls, it's vital to focus on balance, flexibility, and strength. Falls can be particularly damaging to the elderly because the risk of serious injury is much higher in this population. However, research shows that exercise can reduce the risk of falls by up to 23%.

Some of the best exercises for seniors include low-impact exercises to protect joints. These exercises include water aerobics, Pilates, resistance band workouts, walking, and dumbbell workouts (Senior Lifestyle, n.d.).

Children

Children and teens need a good amount of exercise. So it's essential to begin teaching young children that exercise is necessary for good health.

How can we motivate children to be active? Different children, of course, have different needs, so taking the time to understand a child's personality is an excellent place to start. Children that are interested in being active, are coordinated and athletic, and enjoy working with others may benefit from group sports. They may need to try several different sports to see what interests them most (Fitpro, 2020).

Children who are apathetic about exercise or have lower energy levels may need more assistance to get regular activity into their schedules. Parents of these children might need to be more involved in their children's exercise and should lead by example. Getting the whole family to exercise together can be an excellent place to start with children who have these types of personalities. Examples of activities for non-athletes could include shooting hoops in the driveway or running around in the backyard. These activities may be less pressure for children who don't find themselves particularly athletic. Other ideas include games involving physical activity (think Tag or Simon Says), treasure hunts, walking the family dog, or fitness video games like the Nintendo Wii.

Teens

Teens may be resistant to exercise, so it's a good idea to have a plan for incorporating activity into their lives. This plan could mean after-school sports or more casual activities like skateboarding. In addition, parents can support their children in regular exercise by providing transportation and necessary equipment (Gavin, n.d.).

Types of Exercise

What types of exercise are there, and how do we choose? The National Institute on Aging (n.d.) recommends:

Endurance

Endurance, or aerobic activities, increase heart rate and breathing. These types of exercises can improve heart, lung, and circulatory health. When we practice endurance activities, we can continue doing them for longer and longer periods of time. Some classic examples of aerobic activities are running, dancing, swimming, biking, or walking. Some sports may also be considered aerobic, such as soccer, basketball, or tennis.

To safely begin endurance activities, always warm up and cool down. It's also important to ease into these activities as they can cause injuries if our bodies are pushed too much or too quickly. Hydration is essential, as is proper attire for exercising outdoors.

Strength

Muscular strength is vital for building our everyday life skills, such as lifting groceries or climbing stairs. Some people utilize weights to improve strength, but bodyweight exercises such as air squats can be just as effective for beginners. Resistance bands are stretchy bands that can also offer a more challenging workout.

It's vital to incorporate major muscle groups into strength training at least two days per week, but the same muscle groups shouldn't be exercised two days in a row to allow for recovery. We should also aim to balance out the muscles we exercise to avoid making one part of our body stronger than another.

Balance

Balance exercises are essential as we age because this type of exercise can help prevent falls. Examples of balance exercises include yoga, Tai Chi, and standing on one foot.

Flexibility

Flexibility is essential because it makes our everyday activities easier. It should also be used in conjunction with the other exercises above, as it's important to stretch after our muscles are already warmed up. There are stretches for just about every part of the body. Some stretches may also be beneficial for those of us with office jobs, as we may get tightness in our hips and backs from sitting or discomfort in our necks from poor posture.

Now that we've covered the upsides of exercise, let's look at another activity that can be particularly beneficial when it comes to rest: hobbies.

Chapter Six

The relaxing power of a hobby

Neil is 65 years old and fears retirement. He's worked on Wall Street for as long as he can remember and cannot envision himself ever doing any other job. Neil revels in the challenge and bustle of his role and immensely enjoys the variety of tasks for him to do every day. He is an anxious person by nature and finds that he likes to keep busy to preserve his happiness.

Several of Neil's friends have retired in the past few years, and he sees a worrying trend in many of their lives. One of his friends, Matt, worked for the city of New York for many years. Matt's job was the centerpiece of his life and a large part of his identity. Recently, Neil has seen less of Matt. His texts go unanswered, and Matt has been absent from group activities. Finally, Neil decides to visit Matt's apartment, just three blocks away from his home. It's two in the afternoon, and Neil finds Matt sitting in his pajamas on the couch. Matt tells Neil that since retirement, he's not been doing much. Matt finds himself sleeping later into the day, watching TV, and going to bed early. Without his job, Matt feels like he has no purpose anymore.

Neil is shocked by Matt's decline and tells him so. Neil insists that Matt join him in his weekly book club as a start. Reading is a hobby that Neil has had for many years, and he knows Matt also loves reading. Matt's face lights up at the suggestion. When Neil gets up to leave, Matt does too and starts heading towards his closet. "What are you doing?" asks Neil. Matt turns to him with a newfound twinkle in his eye. "I've got to get my sneakers and go get that book right away if I'm going to finish it by our book club on Thursday!"

Why is it important to have a hobby?

Although they may seem trivial, hobbies are actually an important part of life. Hobbies can improve our social lives by allowing us to meet new people and create bonds with others who have similar interests. Additionally, hobbies can make us more interesting and allow us to share our experiences and stories with others. We can also create new connections with people by teaching them the skills we have learned.

Hobbies can assist us with developmental tools like patience and curiosity. If we decide to learn a new hobby, we need to be patient with ourselves during the learning process. In turn, this can help us become more patient with others. Learning something new can challenge us, which may feel uncomfortable at first, but ultimately leads to growth.

Hobbies are distinct in that they differ from both work and passive relaxation. Initially, a hobby may not always be easy, and it might take some effort to learn. This difference distinguishes it from passive relaxation because it sometimes takes mental or physical effort to master it. But a hobby is still pleasurable. Moreover, when we master a new hobby or skill, it can help boost our confidence and self-esteem and make our lives more fulfilling (Skilled at Life, n.d.).

Health benefits of hobbies

Hobbies can help us alleviate mental and physical health concerns. Social prescribing is a treatment method used by medical practitioners who work with depressed patients, particularly patients who suffer from mild to moderate depression. This method suggests that patients take up hobbies or other social endeavors to improve depression symptoms. Because antidepressant medications can be less effective for mild depression, social prescribing may be a good alternative.

Research suggests (The Conversation, 2021) that specific psychological treatments such as social prescribing or behavioral activation (scheduling time to do things that bring pleasure or joy) improve symptoms of depression. The type of activities that have been studied includes gardening, art, exercising, playing an instrument, drawing, reading, or crafts.

These types of treatments are thought to work due to the reward system in the brain. For example, endorphins like dopamine (the feel-good neurotransmitter) are released when we participate in a hobby. These chemicals make us feel happier, kick-start our reward system, and increase our motivation to do the hobby again.

Physical hobbies can improve our fitness, and some hobbies like playing an instrument can improve memory. Additionally, some artistic hobbies like reading or puzzles have been shown to prevent neurological conditions such as dementia later in life. Research has also shown a correlation between physically healthier people (lower body mass index, smaller waists, lower blood pressure, fewer stress hormones, and better overall physical functioning) and people who have hobbies and leisurely pursuits. Although having a hobby does not necessarily cause people to have these healthy traits, it's interesting that there is a strong correlation between the two.

Hobbies can also improve work performance. A study done by researchers at San Francisco State University found that people who had creative pursuits in their personal lives were better at utilizing creative problem-solving at work. This study also found that hobbies gave workers an outlet for recovering from their jobs, increased their sense of control, and often challenged them to learn new skills that could then be transferable to work.

Hobbies and demographics

The U.S. Bureau of Labor Statistics (2015) measures the hours spent on different hobbies by gender, age, and educational attainment.

While men and women tend to be similar in hours spent socializing and thinking, there are marked differences in other activities. For example, women spend more time watching TV and reading, whereas men spend more time playing computer games or sports. These statistics are interesting because they can give insight into each gender's preference. As we know, exercise is one of the best ways to take care of our health, so it may be necessary for women to consider engaging in more sports or recreation activities in their free time. In contrast, men may benefit from positive mental health effects and slower age-related brain issues by engaging in more reading during their leisure time (Lippa, 2005).

When we consider age groups, the elderly tend to engage in more passive hobbies, such as watching tv, thinking, and reading. Unsurprisingly, the youngest age groups tend to engage in the least amount of thinking and most computer games and sports. Socializing and communicating are fairly even among all groups, which is encouraging, as we know that social ties are an essential factor in well-being. Unfortunately, as we age, we tend to engage in less active and more passive activities. It is vital to try and combat this trend, as exercise significantly influences our health.

When considering a participant's education levels, there are more similarities in hobbies than we might think (less than a high school diploma, high school graduates, some college, and bachelor's degree and higher). All groups are about even when it comes to socializing, computer games, and sports. When it comes to passive activities, the more educated we get, the less TV we watch. Interestingly, while the highest education group engages in the most reading, the lowest level education group engages in the most thinking in their spare time.

Hobbies vs. interests

When we begin choosing a hobby, it's crucial to differentiate hobbies and interests.

Interests are general desires to learn about something new. This interest can come from natural curiosity, family history, or professional goals. An example of this would be an interest to know more about football because your significant other enjoys watching games on Sundays. Unlike hobbies, interests only require intellectual action, but not physical action.

Hobbies are defined as enjoyable activities that we do voluntarily when free from other responsibilities. Hobbies can be inspired by interests, but they generally require more commitment. Hobbies are more of an active pursuit and involve taking physical action, like building or creating something (Parker-Pope, n.d.)

How to make time for a hobby

The American Time Use Survey (U.S. Bureau of Labor Statistic, n.d.) is a tool used to measure the amount of time Americans with full-time jobs spend doing various activities throughout their day:

- Household chores: 0.96 hours (This is an average. When we look at gender differences, men spend 49 minutes on chores, whereas women spend 80 minutes)

- Eating/drinking: 1.11 hours

- Leisure/sports: 3.04 hours (This is also an average. Men spend 3.5 hours in this category, whereas women spend 2.3 hours)

- Sleeping/personal care: 8.64 hours

- Caregiving (for parents and children): 0.53 hours

- Shopping: 0.43 hours

- Working: 8.8 hours

So, looking at this jam-packed day, how can we find time to squeeze in a hobby as well? It may benefit us to look at our time differently. Rather than thinking about time in days, it can be more helpful to look at it in terms of weeks. An excellent way to do this is to try tracking a week of your life through traditional pen and paper or an app or calculator.

After tracking our time, many of us might be surprised to find we have more free time than we initially thought. Our perceptions of how much time we have may not match the reality because much of our downtime is spent doing mindless tasks like checking email, scrolling through social media, or using the internet. People with tiring jobs (i.e., most of us) tend to come home and "crash" at the end of the day, which can add up to a lot of lost time doing nothing but recuperating. Participating in hobbies is more effective than complete vegetation to help preserve mental health.

Another vital factor to consider when thinking about time is that too much free time is actually detrimental. One study found that having too much idle time causes us to be just as unhappy as not having enough. For people with full-time jobs, the sweet spot of downtime is 2.5 hours per day. However, for those who are retired or unemployed, the most beneficial amount of time is 4.75 hours per day.

Should we schedule our free time? Research shows that successful people plan their weekends in advance, but they do not overschedule. For example, people planned "anchor events" but were not too rigid about the details surrounding them because overscheduling causes our brains to equate this with work, and thus, we enjoy events less (Parker-Pope, n.d.).

Screens and hobbies

At the end of a busy week, many people prefer to slump down on the comfortable couch and watch TV. However, research shows that binge-watchers get poorer sleep because screens stimulate us physiologically and psychologically. Utilizing screens as hobbies also tends to isolate us more from the people we love, so it's a good idea to prioritize hobbies that do not require screens when possible (Jay Higgins, n.d.).

How to pick a hobby

Where should we begin when thinking about how to pick a hobby? It can be helpful to ask ourselves some questions and even write down the answers. Here are some starter questions:

What is something you've always wanted to do? Think back to conversations you've had with friends or family. Have you ever started a sentence with "I've always wanted to..."? A hobby can be something you've always thought about pursuing but never actually went through with for one reason or another.

What did you like to do as a child? A good place for inspiration is our childhood. Did you participate in sports or clubs after school? Were you called to painting or drawing? Did you love putting on plays for your parents or reading them the stories you invented? Our true selves can often be found in our inner children.

How do you like to spend your time? If you utilize one of the "free time calculators" found online, you can see how you spend most of your time outside of work. For example, the "cooking" section of the pie chart may be quite large for some of us. This piece of information can indicate that you enjoy cooking, as you tend to spend more time on it. Other pursuits to consider include being outdoors, taking photos, reading, or playing with your pet. These things can all serve as inspirations for new hobbies.

Another way of finding a hobby may be to immerse yourself in new or unfamiliar situations. By experiencing new activities like going to a concert, visiting a museum, or even walking around a craft store, we can see what we enjoy doing. Trying out a class or lesson can also be helpful to learn about your passions and spark new ideas.

Alternatively, we can look to everyday activities for inspiration. Activities that are required of us may lead to exciting hobbies. Some examples include:

Cooking: Many of us spend hours a week cooking for ourselves, meal-prepping, or feeding our families. Although this may seem more like a chore, it's possible that we also enjoy it a little. This activity can become more fun by reframing it as a hobby or explorative activity. Cooking classes are a good start, as they can be more fun than cooking alone. We can also learn new technical skills like baking and decorating an intricate cake or making the perfect souffle.

Pets: If you love spending time with your pet, this can give some insight into a possible new hobby. Animal shelters are always looking for volunteers, so this may be something to explore. For those of us that are retired, raising and training service dogs can also be an option. Although this hobby is a significant commitment, it can also be immensely fulfilling. A lower commitment activity would be dog training classes to teach your friend new tricks, or offer to do dog walking in your neighborhood!

Driving kids to activities: Although this particular chore may seem unappealing, it can also spark our own adult hobbies. If we find ourselves immersed in children's sports or clubs, we may also be able to see some joy and find some interest there. For example, creating new uniforms for a sports team or updating a club website might be a potential hobby.

Exercise can also act as a hobby! Runners can join running groups in their neighborhoods to help with accountability and make new friends. Yoga is an excellent hobby because it's easy for anyone to pick up. Strength training generally requires equipment and a coach when starting out but can lead to participation in competitions. Finally, meditation (this will be covered more fully in the next chapter) can also act as a hobby for our minds (Komar & Wylde, 2021).

How hobbies can improve our careers

Having hobbies can also help us be more productive and happier at work. One study published in the Journal of Occupational and Organizational Psychology (Ward, 2017) found that people who engage in creative hobbies in their free time have more positive work-related traits such as better attitudes and increased creativity on work projects. Research also shows that those with hobbies are more satisfied with their jobs and have a lower likelihood of burnout.

As we know, hobbies can improve our mental health. It can increase focus, improve happiness, and lead to longer lives. These benefits are helpful as they relate to work behaviors because they can extend hours or even days following. In addition, the lowered levels of depression and negative feelings can carry over into our workday, and over time this can lead us to be happier in our careers in the long run.

How to Find (Physical) Space for your New Hobby

Tricia is a corporate executive who recently discovered a love of painting. After being encouraged by her wife, Katie, to pursue something new, she tried out several different art forms before landing on painting. She loves the freedom of transforming a blank canvas and finds calm and catharsis when she dips her brushes into globs of new paint.

Once Tricia decided that painting would be her new hobby, she went out and purchased an easel, a basic 12 pack of acrylic paint, and 3 brushes. However, in the following months, she found herself adding more and more to her collection. She now owns 14 brushes of varying sizes and shapes, a standing easel, a small lap easel, and her paint collection has increased exponentially. As a result, Katie has become frustrated with her, as her supplies have spread throughout the house. Tricia often paints in the dining room, her brushes and paper covering the table, so she's beginning to think she may need to come up with a new organizational system before her hobby gets too out of control.

When we discover a new hobby, we may need certain equipment to participate. For example, if we get into a creative hobby like art, we may need paintbrushes, an easel, tarp, palettes, and a smattering of other items. Some people may find the idea of buying new equipment and finding a place to store all of it daunting. Here are some tips for dealing with this potential issue (Parker-Pope, n.d.):

Create a space for your hobby. If you have an extra room in your home that can be repurposed, that can be an easy solution for keeping it organized. If a whole room is not available, you can consider an organization tool of some kind, like a trunk, closet, cabinet, shelf, or drawer. Having a space where all of your equipment is stored can make it easier to transition into your new hobby. Rather than hunting all over the house for materials, a dedicated space can ensure you're able to hop right into creativity.

Keep it organized. Once a space has been allocated, it's a good idea to create a system that works for you. Craft stores like Michael's often have art-specific organization tools, whereas more extensive hardware or general stores can offer organizational systems for other types of equipment. Label makers can help you to access often-used items quickly, and bins, baskets, or jars can keep all of your tools in one place.

Make it easy to access. One barrier to building a hobby habit can be ease of access. If you are constantly searching for things that you need for your hobby, you're less likely to engage in the hobby. For example, if your hobby is exercise, you should be able to find your sneakers, yoga mat, or water bottle in a cinch. The longer it takes to find your materials, the less likely you are to engage in the hobby.

Don't get too sentimental. If you decide on a hobby where you'll be creating something new, like artwork or pottery, you may initially find yourself struggling to decide what to do with your creations. These decisions can lead to a pile of work sitting in the corner that grows and grows. When starting a new creative hobby, it's vital to recognize that you may not be great at it immediately, and that's okay! That being said, you may not need to keep all of your early creations, or even any of them. To remember what you've made, you might consider taking photos of the work and then discarding or repurposing your creations so they don't start to take over too much of your workspace.

Be selective. If your hobby includes collecting things, you'll want to ensure you are particular about what you decide to keep. For example, if you collect baseball cards and find yourself with hundreds of albums, it may be a good idea to pare down your collection to only the most important or valuable cards. What is "valuable" to you may be completely different from the societal definition, so it's helpful to look inward to understand how you define the word. You may prize the items worth the most money, or alternatively, the cheapest items to which you have the most emotional connection. In the end, if you decide to part ways with some of your things, you could consider selling them or donating them.

Go minimal. When you get a new hobby, you might initially buy lots of tools you end up not needing or not using much. Every few months, it's a good idea to take an inventory of your supplies and see what you use often and what can be discarded. If these items are in good condition and could be reused, consider donating them to local teachers or charity shops. Another way to limit the amount of "stuff" you need for your hobby can be to choose a hobby that doesn't require too many physical supplies. Some examples of these types of hobbies include running, theater, or language lessons.

Limit your hobbies. Hobbies should be special to you, so it makes sense not to take on too many at once. Humans can only focus on so many things before they find themselves to be spread too thin, so it's essential to be intentional about how you choose to spend your time. Although it's okay to try out a few different hobbies initially, it's recommended that you whittle it down to just one or two so you can spend quality time participating and engaging.

Now that we've looked at the importance of hobbies, let's turn to meditation and mindfulness to understand how we can be purposeful and present in our lives.

Chapter Seven

Meditation and Mindfulness

Origin and definition

In Western cultures, meditation has become more popular in the past few years. Let's look at the origins of the practice to understand it better. The origins of meditation are debated by scholars, as meditation shows up in several historical records from different cultures like Hinduism, Taoism, Buddhism, and Judaism (Mead, 2021).

India

Meditation is believed to have originated several thousand years ago in India. The word "meditate" comes from the Latin word meditatum, which means "to ponder". In India, the oldest written records from 1500 BCE reference "Dhyana" or "Jhana", which discuss the training of the mind.

In India, Vendatism is a school of philosophy that focuses on paths for spiritual enlightenment. This philosophy is thought to be one origin of meditation from 1500 BCE. The Vedas described meditative practices in their texts, although many of these were passed down for centuries through oral storytelling.

In addition to Vedic practice, Hindu traditions reference the Yogi practice of cave meditation. Modern practices of meditation and yoga stem from this tradition.

Also, in India, Buddhism includes references to the Pali Canon in the 1st century BCE, which describes different states of meditations. Buddha was a prince who then became a monk, philosopher, and religious leader. He taught many people his practices of meditation and founded the Buddhist religion.

Jainism is another form of teaching that places a strong emphasis on self-discipline and non-violence. Jainism utilizes mantras and visualizations and encourages a focus on breathing.

China

In China, meditation is referenced as far back as the 3rd and 6th century BCE in writings by Lao-Tze, an ancient Chinese philosopher whose name translates to "Old Teacher" or "Old Master". However, scholars are unsure whether Lao-Tze was a single man or a collection of philosophers with similar ideas. His writings describe meditation techniques such as "Shou Zhong" (guarding the middle), "Bao Yi" (embracing the one), "Shou Jing" (guarding tranquility), and "Bao Pu" (embracing simplicity). In addition, he is credited with creating Taoism, which emphasizes becoming one with Tao, which means "cosmic life" or "nature".

Lao-Tze is credited for writing the Tao-te-Ching, a text that laid the groundwork for the philosophy of Taoism and referenced wisdom in silence and meditative practices. Traditional Taoist meditation techniques focus on mindfulness, contemplation, and tools such as visualization.

Confucius was a philosopher, teacher, and politician in the 6th century BCE. The philosophy of Confucianism is still popular in modern China, and it emphasizes morality, personal growth, and social justice. Self-improvement and contemplation are also encouraged.

Japan

Dosho was a Japanese monk who studied Buddhism in China in the 7th century. There, he learned the art of Zen. Then, Dosho returned to Japan and opened a meditation hall dedicated to sitting meditation or "Zazen". He also taught a community of monks and students in order to spread awareness of, and the practice of meditation in Japanese culture.

Islam

Sufism is an Islamic tradition dating back 1400 years, and it is thought to have developed through Indian influence. In this practice, Muslims seek to connect with Allah (God) through contemplation and self-reflection. This tradition also emphasizes the shunning of material goods, a focus on breathing, and the use of mantras.

Judaism

Judaism references "lascuach" in the holy scripture (the Torah), which is defined as a form of meditation. In addition, the Jewish school of thought called Kabbalah also includes forms of meditation based on deep thoughts about philosophical topics and prayer.

Meditation in the West

According to Mead (2021), in the 1700s, meditation made its way to the West when Eastern philosophy texts were translated into several different European languages. The texts included were the Upanishads, the Buddhist Sutras, and the Bhagavad Gita. The Upanishads are Indian philosophical texts written between 800 and 500 BCE, and the Buddhist Sutras are scriptures thought to be the oral teachings of the Buddha. The Bhagavad Gita is a Hindu epic composed of 700 verses. This Sanskrit scripture details a narrative between a Hindu prince and Krishna.

In the 18th century, meditation was only discussed by philosophers like Voltaire and Schopenhauer, but by the 20th-century, meditation became more prominent among the general population. In the United States, a prominent yogi, Swami Vivekananda, created a presentation and delivered it in Chicago at the Parliament of Religions. This presentation spurred an interest in Eastern models of spirituality. Moreover, it led many other Indian spiritual teachers to migrate to the U.S., including Swami Rama, Paramahansa Yogananda, and Maharishi Mahesh Yogi.

By the 1960s and 70s, meditation had become shaped by Western culture and more disconnected from the religious aspects. Meditation was being researched in scientific studies to understand its potential benefits better. It was also starting to be recommended as a practice that anyone could do. During the '70s, meditation techniques were associated with Hippie culture and were even utilized by The Beatles to help them cope with stresses of fame and fortune.

In 1993, a book called Ageless Body, Timeless Mind was published and featured on Oprah. Celebrities began praising meditation, which helped bring the practice into popular culture. The idea of mindfulness also gained traction as scientists started exploring it as an alternative or complementary option for people suffering from anxiety and depression.

Today, many resources and schools are available for people interested in mindfulness and meditation. Scientists continue to study the benefits of these practices, which we'll cover in the following few sections.

Benefits of MM

Jose recently started dating a yoga instructor, Lilya. Lilya teaches yoga every day in 1-hour classes and has invited Jose to check out her mindfulness class. Jose is hesitant. He's not very flexible! However, Lilya assures him that this particular class is focused more on his mind and less on his body, so he should be just fine.

Jose enters the class after a long day at work. He's tired and frustrated and would rather not be in this room filled with old ladies on mats, but he wants to try the class for Lilya. So he decides to stay and keep an open mind. For an hour, Lilya leads the class through quiet mindfulness meditation. They practice guided breathing and visualization techniques and pay attention to their bodies.

As Lilya begins to raise the lights at the end of class, Jose notices that his mind is blank. He feels wonderful and calm and can't seem to remember why he was so stressed when he entered the room! He slowly returns to a seated position and vows to continue his mindfulness (with Lilya's help, of course).

Mental

Numerous studies have looked at the mental benefits of meditation and mindfulness. For example, one study found that expert meditators outscored their peers and younger participants in a visual attention test.

Another study in Amsterdam had both novice and expert meditators complete a three-month meditation retreat where participants meditated for 20 minutes per day. At the end of the retreat, the experts outperformed the novices in attention tasks, which points to higher brain efficiency in people who meditate regularly.

Meditation can also strengthen and improve our brain structures (Jabr, 2013). Over time, meditators show a more wrinkled cortex (the brain's outer layer), which is responsible for abstract thinking and introspection. The frontal cortex is also thickened by meditative practice, which helps us to rein in and control our emotions. Meditators also increase the volume and density of their hippocampus, which is responsible for memory and helps reduce the amount of wilting that our brains suffer from as we age.

Scientists are not quite sure how long it takes for meditation to influence our brains, but some experiments suggest that consistent meditation every day for a few weeks can make a difference. In addition, some studies indicate that daily meditation is more important than the total hours of practice over a lifetime. For example, one study on U.S. marines showed that a mere 12 minutes of mindfulness meditation daily helped protect against stressful effects on working memory (Schatz, 2019).

Meditation can also be helpful for people struggling with psychological disorders (Powell, 2018), such as addiction or overeating. Psychologists have utilized mindfulness as an adjunct treatment to help people better understand and tolerate their cravings.

We can utilize this knowledge by injecting mindfulness into small moments of our day. For example, we can try to implement mindfulness techniques on our commutes to work, instead of scrolling on our phones (however, not while driving). On short walks, trading our cell phones for attention to our surroundings can also be a form of meditation. It's essential to become aware of these moments of downtime available to us every day and make the best use of them when possible.

Physical

Mindfulness also has positive physical effects on our bodies (Suttie, 2018).

Heart Health

As we know, heart disease is the number one cause of death in the United States. Studies show that people with prehypertension (high blood pressure) benefit more from mindfulness meditation than muscle relaxation. People with heart disease also show improvements in cardiovascular capacity and slower heart rates after meditation. Mindfulness is also helpful for healthy hearts, as it can increase natural variations in our heart rates, indicating increased survival rates of heart attacks.

Cognition

As we age, we can lose our short-term memory and cognitive flexibility. As we discussed in the previous section, mindfulness meditation can increase attention. Studies on people with

Alzheimer's disease show significant improvement in cognitive scores after meditation.

Immune System

Mindfulness meditation has been shown to increase the levels of T-cells (immune cells that help fight disease) in our bodies. T-cells are necessary for fighting diseases like cancer and HIV. Meditation has also been shown to speed up wound healing.

Cell Aging

As we age, our cells also age and divide. Proteins called telomeres protect our cells from aging. Telomeres can be lengthened, and their activity can be changed by meditation. Although there is not yet much specific data on this particular mechanism, scientists are optimistic about meditation's effect on aging.

Meditation and Therapy

As meditation has become more mainstream, therapists and psychologists have begun integrating it into their practices (Harvard Medical School, 2014). Because meditation focuses on attention, self-forgetfulness, and heightened awareness of our bodies, it can be helpful for people who struggle with negative attitudes towards themselves. For example, many people who deal with anxiety and depression are preoccupied with the negative things in their lives, and meditation can help them move towards self-understanding and forgiveness.

There are several ways meditation can be integrated into different psychological models. One type of therapy, Acceptance and Commitment Therapy, focuses on the idea of control as a problem rather than a solution. Many of us try to suppress or avoid bad feelings and thoughts, making matters worse as we are constantly battling ourselves. This type of therapy is helpful as meditation invites us to focus on these feelings rather than avoid them. By focusing on the difficult emotions and thoughts, we form a "truce" of sorts with them, and they lose their power. Acceptance and commitment therapy allows us to view these thoughts more objectively as they float into our consciousness. We acknowledge them and then let them go.

This type of mindfulness therapy can also be helpful to break negative associations we may have formed over time. For example, a patient who has recovered from depression may struggle with any feelings of general sadness, self-deprecation, or frustration because they have associated these feelings with clinical depression. This struggle may lead to a downward spiral that can exacerbate our negative emotions and another depressive episode. To combat this, therapists can use mindfulness meditation to encourage patients to notice mood changes when they break the cycle of depressive thinking. By helping patients disengage from these thoughts, they can observe them objectively through an attitude of "detached kindly curiosity" and then let them come and go without weight.

Silent Retreats

Silent retreats are getaways that offer long stretches of meditation time and quiet. Although some of these experiences can be quite expensive, there are also many more affordable retreats, and they often include room and board.

Silent retreats can empty our brains so we can relish in silence. This silence can help us become more mindful of our surroundings and truly allow our brains to relax. We are also better able to notice the beauty of nature and cultivate gratitude. In addition, retreats often forbid the use of technology, so they can also act as a disconnection from the reliance that many of us have on our devices.

Silent retreats may allow us to get a sense of the environments that our brains and nervous systems were designed for, considering the types of environments where our ancestors lived. Hours of quiet nothingness can sound quite boring, but they also allow us to return to a time when things were simpler. Because our ancestors dealt with long stretches of quiet and sameness, our brains also evolved to seek out novel experiences. We now live in an environment with an endless supply of new stimuli available 24/7 in our pockets. Through silent retreats, people can allow their brains to have a break from stimuli and return to a resting state (Taft, 2011).

How to meditate

So, after learning about all of the benefits of meditation, how can we actually do it? Of course, meditation is an individual experience and may look different for everyone, but here are some general tips for beginning the meditative practice (Mindful, n.d.):

1. *Sit down.* Meditation is easier to practice in a calm and quiet place. Sitting is more manageable than standing for humans during long periods, so it's recommended for more effortless practice.

2. *Set a time limit.* For beginners, it's essential to set a limit for practice. The time limit can be short, even just 5 or 10 minutes.

3. *Notice the body.* Get into a comfortable sitting position for you. This position could mean crossed legs, kneeling, sitting on the floor, or a chair. Whichever position is chosen, make sure it is stable and can be maintained for some time.

4. *Feel the breath.* Notice the sensation of breathing as it enters and exits the lungs.

5. *Notice the mind.* The attention will invariably stray from the breathing process as a new meditator. When this happens, simply notice it happened and return the attention to the breathing.

6. *Be kind.* As a new meditator, it can be hard not to judge ourselves for our wandering minds. Try to be gentle and return your focus to the breathing.

7. *Close with kindness.* When the timer is up, gently bring back attention to the environment. Notice the sounds nearby and how the body is feeling. Notice any thoughts and emotions that may have come up.

That's it! As we become more comfortable with meditation, we can extend our practice time. However, it's important to remember to try and meditate regularly, even if it is just for short periods of time. If meditation feels too overwhelming to try without guidance, meditation apps that will guide us step-by-step through the process can also be utilized. Examples of such apps include Headspace and Calm (Greene, 2020).

In the next chapter, we'll take a look at forest bathing and the restorative effects of nature.

Chapter Eight

Forest bathing and the healing power of nature

Allie is a stressed-out 32-year-old with multiple jobs. She's been in therapy for many years and has tried every antidepressant under the sun. She recently moved to a new city, and her new therapist seems promising, if not a little "hippy-dippy" for her tastes. However, Allie is a thorough person and believes in science-backed approaches and theories, so she is skeptical when her therapist brings up the idea of "ecotherapy". Her therapist senses this and suggests Allie research the topic and report back.

After some reading, Allie discovers that ecotherapy has been around for quite a long time and has been shown to have many mental and physical benefits. Her therapist suggests she look into forest bathing and give it a try. Allie commits to the endeavor one weekend and fully immerses herself in nature. She is surprised to find that she feels a sense of restoration and peace that hasn't been present in a long time. She decides to continue therapy with an added dose of nature.

In this chapter, we'll take a look at the benefits of nature as they relate to our well-being. We'll cover the physical and psychological benefits, as well as strategies for increasing our exposure to nature.

What are ecotherapy and ecopsychology?

The origins of ecopsychology and ecotherapy can be traced back to the 1960s. It is connected to several scientists and philosophers, including Robert Greenway, Paul Shephard, Theodore Roszak, and Ralph Metzner. The principles of ecopsychology include reciprocity between humans and nature, healing through the environment, and ethical responsibility to the planet. In a nutshell, "the needs of the planet are the needs of the person, the rights of the person are the rights of the planet."

From ecopsychology, ecotherapy was born. Ecotherapy focuses on the environmental and ecological benefits of counseling modalities. Ecotherapy is based on the idea that there is a mutually beneficial relationship between the planet and humans, and through this relationship, people can heal their mental and physical health. Practices of ecopsychology include the appreciation of nature, interacting with animals, therapeutic farming, and nature arts and crafts. Ecopsychology is based on the symbiotic relationship between people and the environment. As people engage in conservation efforts, the planet is restored and imparts those benefits back onto the people (Summer & Vivian, 2018).

Forest Bathing

A subset of ecotherapy is forest bathing, from the Japanese "Shinrinyoku". Forest bathing involves immersing oneself in the forest for a specific amount of time to promote rest and relaxation.

Several studies have shown the beneficial effects of forest bathing. These include a decrease in blood glucose and blood pressure in people with diabetes (McEwan, 2021). Additionally, the stress hormone cortisol can be reduced by forest bathing. Forest bathing has also been shown to support the immune system through increasing natural killer cells responsible for tumor cell death. This discovery could have profound effects in cancer research (Li et al., 2007).

So how can we get the benefits of forest bathing? Here are some tips for having the best experience possible:

- The first step is to decide if you want a guide. Many people feel more comfortable in the forest under the guidance of a certified professional. You can find a professional through the Association of Nature and Forest Therapy Guides. If you decide to go alone, follow basic safety practices.

- Next, you'll want to decide what to wear and pack. It's best to choose a moderate weather day, not too hot or cold. Dress in comfortable clothing and sturdy shoes to match the terrain you'll be visiting. It's a good idea to bring a small pack with water, snacks, sunscreen and a hat.

- Choosing the right place to forest bathe is also essential. The denser the forest is, the greater the benefits, but any natural area with trees will suffice. Some other properties to look for include a quiet atmosphere, beautiful scenery, and a good smell. It's important to note that forest bathing is not hiking, so ideally, the area should be mostly flat and easy to walk on.

- Please turn off your electronic devices and store them in your pack to minimize distractions. Engaging your senses is very important for forest bathing, and electronics can distract you from this. Listen to the sounds, look at the scenery, breathe slowly and smell the fragrances of nature. You can even touch the trees, leaves, and soil. Walk slowly to take in everything around you, and feel free to stop every once in a while to sit or look up (Prelle, 2018).

Health benefits from spending time in nature

There has been some research into the physical and mental health benefits of spending time in nature, although this field of science is still growing. Nevertheless, early studies suggest that nature can help us in several ways (Chaudhury & Banerjee, 2020; Song et al., 2021):

Medical Recovery

Viewing nature has been shown to help patients recovering from surgery. For example, one study of patients after gallbladder surgery showed that patients who had a view of nature through their window recovered faster than those who had no window or no natural view.

Patients with flowering plants and foliage in their recovery rooms have more positive emotions and physiological responses (heart rate, fatigue, pain ratings), and require less postoperative medications.

It might be important to think about the implications of this research in our own lives. For example, if we are healing from an injury, or experiencing pain, exposure to nature can be beneficial. Adding plants to our homes can also be an easy way to increase positivity and help our moods.

Pain Reduction

Patients exposed to images of nature are more likely to switch from stronger to weaker pain medication during their recovery period and report less anxiety. Patients can also benefit from nature sounds when combined with natural images. Studies suggest that patients report an increased pain tolerance and threshold. Increased levels of sunlight exposure are also helpful in reducing pain, stress, and the use of painkillers in post-surgical patients.

PTSD

Post Traumatic Stress Disorder (PTSD) is a mental health disorder often resulting from serious trauma. Symptoms include severe anxiety, flashbacks to traumatic events, and hypervigilance (constantly assessing for potential threats in your environment). Many veterans suffer from PTSD.

Some beneficial therapeutic strategies for veterans with PTSD include outdoor adventure activities, wilderness therapy, and green space-based ecotherapy (interactions and participation in nature). Green space therapy is an approach that increases interaction and engagement with green space and has been associated with increased length of life and decreased risk of mental illness. Wilderness therapy is a more structured approach that combines traditional therapeutic techniques and physical activities within nature.

Stress Reduction

Horticultural Therapy (HT) is a rehabilitative strategy involving gardening, interactions with plants, and closeness to nature. HT has been shown to improve mood state through stress reduction, improve self-esteem, reduce depression and improve sleep and cognitive issues in patients with dementia.

Adventure-based nature programs are often used to help adolescents with self-esteem, mood modification, and behavioral issues related to schizophrenia. These programs are usually done in groups, and they encourage teamwork and communication by overcoming natural obstacles. Examples include rock climbing and outdoor ropes courses. Adventure-based treatments have helped mentally ill patients increase their coping skills and have been shown to improve adjustment to brain injury. Additionally, this type of therapy has been shown to help adolescents deal with family trauma and well-being, as well as chemical dependency.

For children living in rural areas, exposure to nature reduced stress and helped children recover faster from stressful events. This result could be due to enhanced coping mechanisms or some combination of social and environmental factors.

ADHD

Attention Deficit Hyperactivity Disorder (ADHD) is a mental health disorder often diagnosed in children. Symptoms include difficulty paying attention, increased hyperactivity, faster than usual speech, and many other negatively affecting a child's interpersonal relationships and personal growth. In addition, current medications for ADHD can have negative side effects, including appetite suppression and sleep disruption, so it may be helpful to look into natural remedies as a complementary treatment.

Several studies suggest that children with ADHD may benefit from increased exposure to green spaces. Motor ability, concentration, and social play are all positively influenced after nature exposure, and symptoms of ADHD have been reduced. It should be noted that adults also perform better on objective attention measures after viewing or spending time in nature.

Dementia

For older adults living in a care facility, exposure to nature can support sensory stimulation and have positive effects. Horticultural therapy may be particularly beneficial for dementia patients that can participate, as it increases their exposure to nature while also promoting engagement and agency. Exposure to nature may also decrease agitation in patients with late-stage dementia.

Obesity

As of 2017, more than 36% of adults and 17% of children in the United States were classified as obese. Obesity is connected to a wide range of health issues, including heart disease, stroke, osteoarthritis, diabetes, and some cancers.

The connection between physical activity and environmental factors is complex and nuanced. For example, people with easy access to nature are less likely to be obese or dependent on antidepressants. In addition, increased green space is associated with reduced weight. In Europe, one study showed that people were 40% less likely to be obese in the greenest areas of eight major cities. These findings may be something to consider when moving to a new location.

Cognitive Benefits of Nature

Nature can help our brains through a variety of mechanisms. One study focused on Attention Restoration Theory (ART), suggests that attention is split into two components: involuntary and voluntary attention. Involuntary attention is attention captured by intriguing or important stimuli, whereas voluntary attention is directed by cognition. An example of involuntary attention would be a fascinating stimulus, such as a sunset, whereas an example of voluntary attention would be choosing to read and then focusing on the book. In this study, researchers had one group of participants walk in nature or view natural scenes while the other group walked downtown in a city or viewed city scenes. The group that interacted with nature physically or visually performed significantly better during voluntary attention tasks than the city group, suggesting that our focused attention can be improved by brief natural exposure.

Studies also show that psychological relaxation effects are improved after exposure to nature. The most beneficial type of exposure seems to be combined visual and auditory natural stimuli, so immersing oneself in nature is the easiest way to improve psychological relaxation. Tactile exposure is also helpful. For example, one study compared cypress wood to touching marble and found that wood exposure improved relaxation.

Virtual reality has also been studied, and results show that participants exposed to a simulation of combined auditory and visual natural scenes exhibit a decrease in the stress hormone cortisol (Berman et al., 2009).

How can nature help us switch off in this digital age?

Researchers at UC Berkeley studied the disconnect between modern life and nature. They found that nature features significantly less in popular culture today than it did in the first half of the 20th century (Kesebir, S. & Kesebir, P., 2017). After the 1950s, mentions of nature steadily declined in popular songs and fiction books. Comparatively, the appearance of words related to human-made environments has not decreased.

One theory for this change is the technological advancement that began in the 1950s. For example, television became the most popular entertainment medium in the 1950s, video games appeared in the 1970s, and the internet has dominated since the late 1990s.

Today, we are inundated with technology and cannot escape it. Understanding the inverse relationship between nature and technology can be helpful in order to take steps to combat it. It is important to take purposeful actions to disconnect ourselves from technology in favor of nature or even utilize technology to get more nature in our lives. Examples of this include watching nature videos (or even having them on in the background) and playing nature sounds while working.

Nature at work

Jayne is an office worker who spends most of her day at the computer. Her cubicle is small, and the office has no windows. Therefore, Jayne prioritizes getting outside every day, during her 15-minute break or 30-minute lunch. Jayne has been following this routine for the past three years while she's worked for the company and finds getting outside helps her power through the afternoon slog.

Jayne hasn't been getting outside in the past few months due to her pregnancy. She finds herself struggling to walk as her belly grows. Lately, she's taken to reading and eating at her cubicle during breaks and lunch. She's noticed her mood declining and finds that her quality of work is not as good as it once was. She chalks this up to pregnancy hormones and hopes it'll pass. Her husband Jeremy suggests that getting outside during the day might help, even if she cannot walk long distances. So one Monday, when her break rolls around, she walks out and sits on a bench in the sun. That afternoon, her productivity feels sky-high, and she finds herself happily chatting with her coworkers. She vows to go outside each day, even just to take a break and soak in some rays on her favorite bench.

How can we utilize nature when we are at work? One study suggests that viewing green spaces can help restore and boost attention. For example, after just 40 seconds of viewing a green roof scene, participants made fewer omission errors in an attention task than participants who viewed a concrete roof (Lee et al., 2015).

As we discussed earlier in this book, microbreaks are helpful in attention restoration, but utilizing these microbreaks in conjunction with nature can be even more beneficial. Researchers suggest that benefits can result even from computer wallpapers or screensavers of nature scenes.

Other research shows that park walks during lunch breaks significantly impact workers' concentration and result in less strain in the afternoon. This study had participants go on a 15-minute park walk during their workday. The results found that spending time in natural environments can restore attentional resources and improve recovery from stress (Sianoka et al., 2018).

Strategies for Incorporating Nature into Everyday Life

So how can we get more nature in our busy lives? Here are some things to consider:

Utilize Weekends

Many of us work 9-5 jobs and don't have much time (or sunlight) to get out into nature during the week. One option for combatting this is to plan nature time for the weekend. If there is a forest or green space nearby, it may be beneficial to plan weekend outdoor time. This plan could simply mean a walk in the park with loved ones or involve a more adventurous activity like hiking or camping.

Maximize Indoor Environments

An easy way to incorporate more nature into our indoor environments is to get houseplants for our homes or offices. Many great indoor plants don't need too much sunlight, and as noted above, plants can promote mental well-being and relaxation. Alternatively, a patio or balcony can be outfitted with hanging plants or succulents that need lots of light. If taking care of a plant seems like too much work, even pictures or posters of nature (maybe one take at a previous holiday) have shown to be beneficial. These images can go on the walls of our homes or become our phone backgrounds or computer screensavers. Nature sounds can also be brought indoors. Consider purchasing a white noise machine that offers birdsong, rain sounds, or ocean waves.

Take Breaks

As we've discussed throughout this book, taking breaks is essential to our well-being. Even just a five-minute break from work or school is beneficial to our health. If this break can be taken in nature, that's an excellent option. Consider walking to nearby green spaces such as parks, or even just take a moment to look up at the sky or close your eyes and hear bird sounds.

In this chapter, we covered the benefits of nature. Next, let's look at how we can combine these strategies with breathing techniques for maximum wellness.

Chapter Nine

Breathing - Take a deep breath

What happens in our bodies when we breathe?

Why do we breathe? Let's look at what happens physiologically when we breathe (National Heart, Lung, and Blood Institute, n.d.). Our lungs are organs that have a spongy texture and a pinkish-gray color. When we inhale, air enters the lungs, and oxygen from the air moves from the lungs into the blood. Simultaneously, carbon dioxide (a waste gas) is transported from the blood into the lungs and is exhaled. This process is known as gas exchange and is essential to all life.

In addition to this process, the respiratory system is responsible for breathing and gas exchange. This system includes the trachea (windpipe), chest muscles in the chest wall, diaphragm, blood vessels, and tissues. Our brains control our breathing rate by sensing the body's need for oxygen and its need to get rid of carbon dioxide.

To promote healthy lungs and prevent lung injuries and diseases, it is vital to get regular exercise, abstain from smoking, and engage in healthy eating habits.

How can anxiety and other mental health issues affect our breathing?

Phyllis is a 40-year-old mom with three children, and she has been suffering from some odd symptoms lately. She finds herself doing ordinary tasks, such as washing the dishes, when suddenly she feels like she cannot breathe. Her heart feels like it is beating too fast, her breathing feels irregular and difficult, and her thoughts start to race. She knows that asthma runs in her family and begins to wonder if that might be what's going on. Her sister, Elise, is concerned about her and insists they go to the ER.

Once they see the doctor, Phyllis begins to describe her symptoms. She makes sure to say that there is a history of asthma in her family, in case this is important for the doctor to know. Instead, her doctor asks if she has a history of anxiety disorders in her family. Phyllis is thrown and immediately says no. Elise suddenly speaks up and says, "Our mother worried all the time but was never diagnosed with anything. She would sometimes have to breathe into a paper bag to calm down." The doctor tells Phyllis that she may be suffering from panic attacks. Phyllis does not want to take medication, but the doctor assures her that there are various ways to treat her symptoms. They discuss breathing exercises, and she makes a referral for Phyllis to see a therapist specializing in anxiety disorders.

When we constantly feel stressed, anxiety and other mental health issues can be exacerbated. Anxiety disorders are some of the most common mental health problems in much of the population, affecting more than 25 million people. It is important to distinguish anxiety disorders from normal anxiety related to stressful events or difficult life situations. For example, people with anxiety disorders have high levels of dread that come out of nowhere, unprovoked. Fight or flight responses may be skewed.

Anxiety disorders can also affect our breathing processes (Ceurstemont, 2020). Interoception is the concept of sensing signals from internal organs. An example of this could be noticing an increased heart rate or the feeling of hunger. Research suggests that people with high anxiety levels may not accurately perceive what's happening inside their bodies. As a result, those with anxiety disorders are less sensitive to changes in their breathing than healthy people. This lack of perception can be a cyclical problem because dysfunctional interoception can be both a cause and effect of anxiety. For example, an anxious person may not notice breathing changes until they become extreme and feel lightheaded. This symptom can then add to their worry and make them even more anxious.

Some anxiety sufferers may also misinterpret bodily signals that can't be medically explained. For example, if someone with anxiety has a headache and is worried they have a brain tumor, they may become stressed, causing their breathing and heart rate to increase. They may then wrongly interpret these symptoms and use them as evidence of having a brain tumor.

Scientists studying the connection between anxiety disorders and breathing are attempting to develop complementary treatments. These treatments may include educating the patient about the relationship between anxiety and breathing and the dysfunctional mechanisms and insight that many anxiety patients suffer.

Health benefits of breathing exercises:

What are the health benefits of breathing exercises? According to Silverton (2020):

1. Improved Immunity – Breathing exercises are helpful because they increase the amount of oxygen in the body and promote the release of toxins. By increasing the amount of oxygen in our cells, our tissues become healthier and perform better. This increase in oxygen also improves our immune system by strengthening our circulatory systems.

2. Taming Anxiety – Deep breathing exercises are often utilized by people who struggle with anxiety. Patients may work with their psychologists to combat panic attacks by focusing on breathing, counting breaths, and other coping techniques. Deep breathing helps bring the heart rate down and helps signal to the brain that there is no threat in the immediate environment.

3. Improved Sleep Quality – Deep breathing can be an excellent way to signal our body to calm down and get ready for sleep. Progressive relaxation exercises combined with deep breathing can be a helpful technique for those who have trouble falling asleep.

4. Decreased Toxicity – Shallow exhalation may promote increased acidity in the body, whereas deep breathing helps balance the body. Deep breathing may also assist in lymphatic drainage.

5. Improved digestion – Breathing techniques increase oxygen in the organs and can help relieve gastrointestinal issues such as constipation and indigestion.

6. Improved Cardiovascular Health – Deep breathing strengthens our cardiovascular muscles and can improve our blood pressure. Diaphragmatic breathing increases lung elasticity and improves lung capacity.

What are some examples of breathing exercises?

There is a variety of breathing techniques. Let's examine some of them:

1. Pursed Lip Breathing – This type of breathing can be 4 to 5 times per day. To practice pursed-lip breathing, inhale slowly through your nose for two counts, then exhale for four counts through pursed lips (imagine you are going to whistle).

2. Diaphragmatic Breathing – This type of breathing, otherwise known as "Belly Breathing", can be done for five to ten minutes at a time. Your diaphragm is located below your rib cage. To practice this type of breathing, begin by laying on your back with your knees slightly bent. Place one hand on your upper chest and one below your rib cage. This position will help you feel the movement of your diaphragm. Slowly inhale through your nose, feeling your stomach pressing into your hand while keeping your other hand as still as possible. Exhale through pursed lips, tighten your stomach muscles and keep your upper hand entirely still.

3. Breath focus technique – This exercise utilizes imagery or focus words. First, you'll want to choose a focus word that works for you, such as "relax" or "peace". You'll want to practice this breathing for ten to twenty minutes. First, sit or lie down in a comfortable place and begin bringing awareness to your breaths. Alternate between regular and deep breaths and notice how your abdomen expands upon deep inhalations. Practice deep breathing for a few minutes, letting out a loud sigh with each exhale. Begin your breath focus by combining your deep breathing with your focus word. Alternatively, you can imagine the air you are inhaling washing away tension and anxiety.

4. Lion's Breath – Lion's breath (or "simhasana" in Sanskrit) is a breathing practice founded in Yoga. To practice this type of breathing, sit on your heels or cross your legs in a comfortable position with your palms flat against your knees and fingers spread wide. Inhale deeply through your nose and open your eyes as wide as you can. Simultaneously open your mouth wide and stick out your tongue, bringing the tip down towards your chin. Contract muscles at the front of your throat while exhaling through your mouth and making a long "ha" sound. Do this breath two or three times.

5. Alternate Nostril Breathing – Alternate nostril breathing (or nadi shodhana pranayama in Sanskrit) has been shown to enhance cardiovascular function and lower heart rate. This type of breathing is most beneficial when done on an empty stomach and with little to no congestion.
First, sit in a comfortable position and lift your right

hand towards your nose to practice this technique. Press your pointer and middle fingers down towards your palm, with your other fingers extended. After an exhale, use your right thumb to close your right nostril gently. Inhale through your left nostril, then close your left nostril with your right pinky and ring fingers. Next, release your thumb and exhale through your right nostril. Then inhale through your right nostril. Continue this process as you feel comfortable.

6. Resonant Breathing – This type of breathing (also known as coherent breathing) has been shown to reduce stress, reduce symptoms of depression (when combined with yoga), and maximize heart rate variability. Simply inhale for a count of five, and exhale for a count of five. Continue the pattern for a few minutes.

7. Sitali Breath – This Yoga breathing technique can help lower body temperature while relaxing the mind. Find a comfortable sitting position, stick out your tongue and curl it to bring the outer edges together. If you can't do this with your tongue, you can purse your lips instead. Next, inhale through the mouth and exhale through the nose. Continue this for up to five minutes.

8. Humming Bee Breath – This breathing practice helps create a sense of calm and can be particularly soothing around the forehead area. In a seated position, close your eyes and relax your face. Place your first fingers on the cartilage that partially covers your ear canal. Inhale, then gently press your fingers to the cartilage as you exhale. Keeping your mouth closed, make a loud humming

sound. Continue this for as long as is comfortable (Cronkleton, 2019; Dr. B. Lal Clinical Laboratory, 2020).

Importance and Benefits of breathing in Yoga

In Yoga, breathing makes up one-half of practice. "Asana" refers to physical posture, whereas "pranayama" means breathing exercises. Pranayama is a Sanskrit word that roughly translates to ideas of the breath of life, vital energy, and expansion of meaning, regulation, and control. Pranayama includes four aspects of breathing, including Puraka (inhalation), Recaka (exhalation), Antah kumbhaka (internal breath retention), and Bahih kumbhaka (external breath retention). Pranayama has been studied in relation to several health issues and seems to have significant benefits:

The effect of pranayama on malignant diseases (such as cancer) has been researched in several studies. Pranayama has been shown to reduce cancer-related fatigue and emotions such as worry, anxiety, frustration, and improvements in sleep. Pranayama has also been shown to improve immune function in cancer patients in remission and increase natural killer cells that fight cancer (Jayawardena et al., 2020).

In patients with cardiovascular diseases, pranayama has been shown to reduce anxiety in patients suffering from heart attacks and patients undergoing surgical procedures. Patients with high blood pressure have also benefited from this practice. Additionally, asthma patients have found relief through pranayama as it is thought to correct abnormal breathing patterns and improve the strength of muscles responsible for inhalation and exhalation.

Pranayama has also been studied in relation to depression symptoms. For example, in one study, battered women utilized pranayama while giving testimony about their abuse. Women in the group that practiced the technique rated lower levels of depressive symptoms than those in the control group (Sutarto et al., 2012).

Breathing on the Job

How can breathing help us to deal with our workplace stressors? As we know, job stress can negatively affect our attention span and memory and may increase anxiety, depression, and the likelihood of burnout. In addition, this job stress can be hazardous in industrial jobs, as it can lead to misjudgment when working with heavy machinery, possibly leading to severe injuries or even death (Sutarto, 2012).

As discussed above, one particularly promising breathing technique is resonant frequency breathing (RFB), where people engage in smooth diaphragmatic breathing. In this technique, respiration rate is essential because it drives our heart rhythm. Biofeedback can be helpful to learn this type of breathing. Biofeedback allows people to connect their physiological indicators (i.e., breathing rate) to audio or visual feedback, so they can more easily regulate their breathing through an improved mind-body connection. Biofeedback and breathing exercises have been shown to help improve many stress-related physical and psychological issues.

One study examined the effect of RFB biofeedback training on manufacturing operators. The levels of occupational stress were measured in terms of anxiety and depression symptoms. After RFB and biofeedback training, the group showed a significant decrease in heartbeats per minute and reduced self-reported anxiety and depression.

The implications of these studies suggest that certain types of breathing while at work can help lower our stress responses and lead to better performance and thus higher job and life satisfaction.

Conclusion

Hopefully, this book has helped you understand the importance of rest and has encouraged you to take some steps to incorporate more of it into your life. By understanding different types of rest, we uncovered its benefits and learned about the physical and mental consequences if we don't get enough of it. We also covered cultural differences when it comes to balancing rest and work and some specific historical events that led to America's current career ideologies. Finally, we've learned many different strategies for integrating and encouraging rest, including exercise, hobbies, reconnecting with nature, and meditation.

I'll leave you with a quote from Thich Nhat Hanh, a global spiritual leader, poet, and peace activist:

"It's very important that we re-learn the art of resting and relaxing. Not only does it help prevent the onset of many illnesses that develop through chronic tension and worrying; it allows us to clear our minds, focus, and find creative solutions to problems."

Thank you for reading!

Thank you for your purchase. If you enjoyed this book, feel free to leave a review on Amazon. This will help us to continue to provide great books, and it will help our potential buyers make confident buying decisions. We will be forever grateful, thank you in advance!

Scan the above QR code, or visit the link below to leave a review:

https://www.rpbook.co.uk/azr/B09W7LFMZR

Alternatively, if you bought the book from Amazon, you can also search for it on your local Amazon store or find it under "your orders" in your Amazon account.

Also by Jessie Fields:

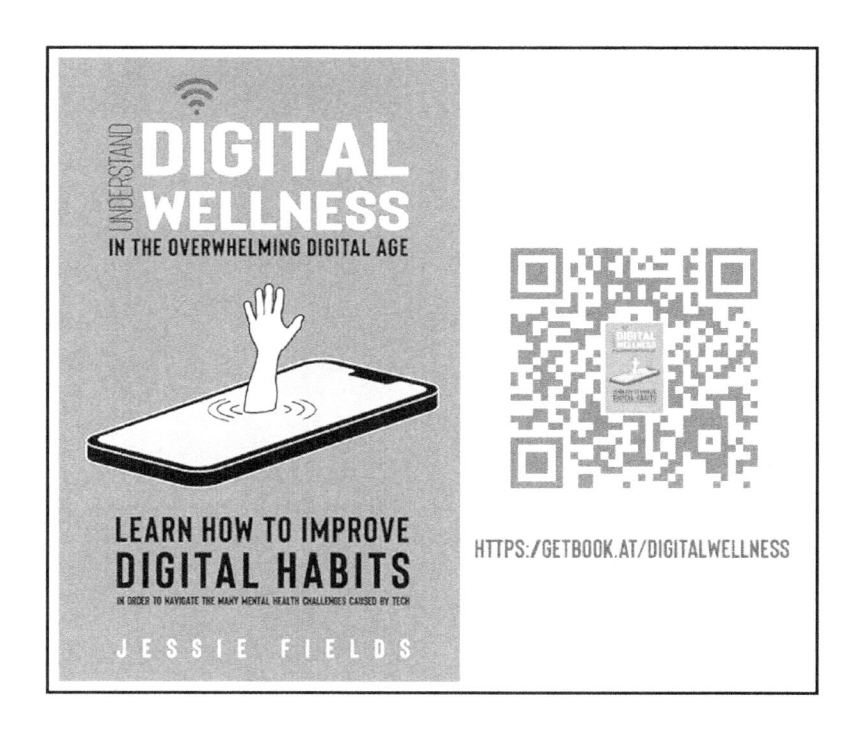

HTTPS:/GETBOOK.AT/DIGITALWELLNESS

References

American Psychological Association. (2018, November 1). *Stress effects on the body.* https://www.apa.org/topics/stress/body

BBC News. (2018, September 15). *Why uganda is the 'world's fittest country'.* https://www.bbc.com/news/world-africa-45496654

Berman, M., Jonides, J., & Kaplan, S. (2009). The cognitive benefits of interacting with nature. *Psychological Science, 19*(12), 1207-1212. 10.1111/j.1467-9280.2008.02225.x

Brenner, B. (2019, September 16). *Creativity is your secret advantage for mental health and well-being.* https://nyctherapy.com/therapists-nyc-blog/creativity-is-your-secret-advantage-for-mental-health-and-well-being/

Briggs, H. (2017, July 12). *Lark or night owl? Blame your ancestors.* BBC news. https://www.bbc.com/news/science-environment-40568997

Brueck, H. (2019, April 23). *Finland and uganda are the world's fittest countries - here's what they do to stay in shape.* Insider.

https://www.businessinsider.com/worlds-fittest-countries-reeal-how-to-stay-in-shape-2019-4

Ceurstemont, S. (2020, June 22). *What anxiety does to our breathing.* Horizon. https://ec.europa.eu/research-and-innovation/en/horizon-magazine/what-anxiety-does-our-breathing

Chang, A., Aeschbach, D., Duffy, J., & Czeisler, C. (2014). Evening use of light-emitting eReaders negatively affects sleep, circadian timing, and next-morning alertness. *PNAS, 112*(4), 1232-1237. https://doi.org/10.1073/pnas.1418490112

Chaudhury, P. & Banerjee, D. (2020). "Recovering with nature": A review of ecotherapy and implications for the COVID-19 pandemic. *Frontiers in Public Health, 8,* 604440. https://doi.org/10.3389/fpubh.2020.604440

Ciulla, J. (2000). *The working life: The promise and betrayal of modern work.* New York: Times Business Books.

Cleveland Clinic. (2019, September 17). *Why exercise protects your brain's health (and what kind is best).* https://health.clevelandclinic.org/why-exercise-protects-your-brains-health-and-what-kind-is-best/

Cleveland Clinic. (2020, June 2). *Why downtime is essential for brain health.* Healthessentials. https://health.clevelandclinic.org/why-downtime-is-essential-for-brain-health/

Cleveland Clinic. (n.d.). *Common sleep disorders.* https://my.clevelandclinic.org/health/articles/11429-common-sleep-disorders

Cohen, S., Janicki-Deverts, D., & Miller, G. (2007). Psychological stress and disease. *JAMA, 298*(14), 1685-1687. 10.1001/jama.298.14.1685

Coleman Wood, K., Lowndes, B., Buus, R., & Hallbeck, M. (2018). Evidence-based intraoperative microbreak activities for reducing musculoskeletal injuries in the operating room. *Work, 60*(4), 649-659. 10.3233/WOR-182772

Colten, H. & Altevogt, B. (Eds.). (2006). *Sleep disorders and sleep deprivation: An unmet public health problem.* National Academies Press.

Cronkleton, E. (2019, April 9). *10 breathing techniques for stress relief and more.* Healthline. https://www.healthline.com/health/breathing-exercise#sitali-breath

Danziger, S., Levav, J., & Avnaim-Pesso, L. (2011). Extraneous factors in judicial decisions. *PNAS, 108*(17), 6889-6892. https://doi.org/10.1073/pnas.1018033108

DiOrio, S. (2019, August 1). *5 ways workplace culture is different around the world.* Viventium. https://www.viventium.com/workplace-culture-around-the-world/

Dr. B. Lal Clinical Laboratory. (2020, November 2). *12 amazing health benefits of breathing exercises.* https://www.blallab.com/blog/12-amazing-health-benefits-of-breathing-exercises/

Egan, C. (2019, August 26). *What is the zeigarnik effect and are you caught up in it?* LinkedIn. https://www.linkedin.com/pulse/what-zeigarnik-effect-you-caught-up-carla-egan-mba-executive/

Falconier, M., Nussbeck, F., Bodenmann, G., Schneider, H. & Bradbury, T. (2015). *Journal of Marital and Family Therapy, 41*(2), 221-235. https://doi.org/10.1111/jmft.12073

Finkbeiner, K., Russell, P. & Helton, W. (2016). Rest improved performance, nature improves happiness: Assessment of break periods on the abbreviated vigilance task. *Consciousness and Cognition, 42,* 277-285. https://doi.org/10.1016/j.concog.2016.04.005

Fitpro. (2020, July 2). *Six fitness ideas for kids who don't like sports.* https://www.fitpro.com/blog/six-fitness-ideas-for-kids-who-dont-like-sports/

Fritz, C. & Sonnentag, S. (2006). Recovery, well-being, and performance-related outcomes: The role of workload and vacation experiences. *Journal of Applied Psychology, 91*(4), 936-945. 10.1037/0021-9010.91.4.936

Gavin, M. (n.d.). *Motivating kids to be active.* KidsHealth. https://kidshealth.org/en/parents/active-kids.html

Greene, P. (2020, November 30). *How long should you meditate for? And how often?* Manhattan Center for Cognitive Behavioral Therapy. https://www.manhattancbt.com/archives/309/how-long-should-you-meditate/#:~:text=Mindfulness%252Dbased%2520clinical%2520interventions%2520such,recommends%252020%2520minutes%252C%2520twice%2520daily

Guttman, J. (2019, December 16). *It's time to declutter and reduce your sensory overload.* Psychology Today. https://www.psychologytoday.com/us/blog/sustainable-life-satisfaction/201912/its-time-declutter-and-reduce-your-sensory-overload

Harvard Medical School. (2007, December 18). *Why do we sleep, anyway?* Healthy sleep. https://healthysleep.med.harvard.edu/healthy/matters/benefits-of-sleep/why-do-we-sleep

Harvard Medical School. (2014, March 9). *Meditation in psychotherapy.* https://www.health.harvard.edu/newsletter_article/Meditation_in_psychotherapy

Harvard Health Publishing. (2020, July 7). *Blue light has a dark side.* Harvard Medical School. https://www.health.harvard.edu/staying-healthy/blue-light-has-a-dark-side

Headversity. (n.d.). *The toxicity of hustle culture: The grind must stop.* https://headversity.com/the-toxicity-of-hustle-culture-the-grind-must-stop/

Helton, W. & Russell, P. (2011). Working memory load and the vigilance decrement. *Experimental Brain Research, 212*(3), 429-437. 10.1007/s00221-011-2749-1

Holstee. (n.d). *Five science-based benefits of journaling.* https://www.holstee.com/blogs/mindful-matter/5-science-based-benefits-of-journaling

Hutson, M. (2012, August 3). Still puritan after all these years. *The New York Times.* https://www.nytimes.com/2012/08/05/opinion/sunday/are-americans-still-puritan.html

Jabr, F. (2013, October 15). *Why your brain needs downtime.* Scientific American. https://www.scientificamerican.com/article/mental-downtime/

Jayawardena, R., Ranasinghe, P., Ranawaka, H., Gamage, N., Dissanayake, D., & Misra, A. (2020). Exploring the therapeutic benefits of pranayama (yogic breathing): A systematic review. *International Journal of Yoga, 13*(2), 99–110. https://doi.org/10.4103/ijoy.IJOY_37_19

Jay Higgins, C. (n.d.). *7 screen-free hobbies to unplug and exercise your creativity.* The Good Trade. https://www.thegoodtrade.com/features/screen-free-hobbies-that-spark-creativity

Kenttä, G. & Hassmén, P. Overtraining and recovery. (1998). *Sports Med, 26,* 1–16. https://doi.org/10.2165/00007256-199826010-00001

Kesebir, S. & Kesebir, P. (2017, September 20). *How modern life became disconnected from nature.* Greater Good Science Center. https://greatergood.berkeley.edu/article/item/how_modern_life_became_disconnected_from_nature

King, A. (2020, December 3). Evolved to run - but not to exercise. *The Irish Times.* https://www.irishtimes.com/news/science/evolved-to-run-but-not-to-exercise-1.4412604

Komar, M. & Wylde, K. (2021, September 16). *11 foolproof ways to find a new hobby.* Bustle. https://www.bustle.com/wellness/how-to-find-hobby-adult

Kuttner, R. (1992, February 2). No time to smell the roses anymore. *The New York Times.* https://archive.nytimes.com/www.nytimes.com/books/business/9806schor-overworked.html?scp=19&sq=robert%252520kuttner&st=cse

Kwok, C., Kontopantelis, E., Kuligowski, G., Gray, M., Muhyaldeen, A., Gale, C., Peat, G., Cleator, J,. Chew-Graham, C., Loke, Y., & Mamas, M. (2018). Self-reported sleep duration and quality and cardiovascular disease and mortality: A dose-response meta-analysis. *J Am Heart Assoc, 7*(15), 1-26. 10.1161/JAHA.118.008552

Lasch, C. (1979). The culture of narcissism: American life in an age of diminishing expectations. W.W. Norton & Company. https://thezeitgeistmovement.se/files/Lasch_Christopher_The_Culture_of_Narcissism.pdf

Lee, K., Williams, K., Sargent, L., Williams, N., & Johnson, K. (2015). 40-second green roof views sustain attention: The role of micro-breaks in attention restoration. *Journal of Environmental Psychology, 42*, 182-189.

https://doi.org/10.1016/j.jenvp.2015.04.003Get

Li, Q., Morimoto, K., Nakadai, A., Inagaki, H., Katsumata, M., Shimizu, T., Hirata, Y., Hirata, K., Suzuki, H., Miyazaki, Y., Kagawa, T., Koyama, Y., Ohira, T., Takayama, N., Krensky, AM., & Kawada, T. (2007). Forest bathing enhances human natural killer activity and expression of anti-cancer proteins. *Int J Immunopathol Pharmacol, 20*(2), 3-8. 10.1177/03946320070200S202

Lippa, R. (2005). How do lay people weight information about instrumentality, expressiveness, and gender-typed hobbies when judging masculinity-femininity in themselves, best friends, and strangers? *Sex Roles, 53*(1-2), 43-55. 10.1007/s11199-005-4277-6

Lufkin, B. (2019, July 21). *Presenteeism.* BBC worklife 101. https://www.bbc.com/worklife/article/20190719-presenteeism

Magnavita, N. & Garbarino, S. (2017). Sleep, health and wellness at work: A scoping review. *International Journal of Environmental Reseach and Public Health, 14*(11), 1347. 10.3390/ijerph14111347

Mayo Clinic. (n.d.). *Sleepwalking.* https://www.mayoclinic.org/diseases-conditions/sleepwalking/symptoms-causes/syc-20353506#:~:text=Sleepwalking%2520%25E2%2580%2594%2520also%2520known%2520as%2520somnambulism,serious%2520problems%2520or%2520require%2520treatment

McEwan, K., Giles, D., Clarke, F.J., Kotera, Y., Evans, G., Terebenina, O., Minou, L., Teeling, C., Basran, J., Wood, W., & Weil, D. (2021). A pragmatic controlled trial of forest bathing compared with compassionate mind training in the UK: Impacts on self-reported wellbeing and heart rate variability.. *Sustainability, 13,* 1380. https://doi.org/10.3390/su13031380

McLean, D., Hurd, A. & Anderson, D. (2019). *Recreation and leisure in modern society.* Jones and Bartlett Publishers. https://samples.jblearning.com/0763749591/49591_ch03_mclean.pdf

Mead, E. (2021, December 14). *The history and origin of meditation.* Positive Psychology. https://positivepsychology.com/history-of-meditation/

Metse, A.., Fehily, C., Clinton-McHarg, T., Wynne, O., Lawn, S., Wiggers, J., & Bowman, J. (2021). Self-reported suboptimal sleep and receipt of sleep assessment and treatment among persons with and without a mental health condition in Australia: a cross sectional study. *BMC Public Health, 21,* (463), 1-12. https://doi.org/10.1186/s12889-021-10504-6

Michel, A. (2016, January 29). *Burnout and the brain.* Association for psychological science. https://www.psychologicalscience.org/observer/burnout-and-the-brain

Milkman, K. & Duckworth, A. (2018, May 1). *Using behavioral science to build an exercise habit.* Scientific American. https://www.scientificamerican.com/article/using-behavioral-science-to-build-an-exercise-habit/

Miller, G. (2020, January 13). *The US is the most overworked developed nation in the world.* 20 Something Finance. https://20somethingfinance.com/american-hours-worked-productivity-vacation/

Miller, J. (2019). *A very brief outline of american labor history for beginners.* California federation of teachers labor and climate justice education committee. https://www.cft.org/sites/main/files/file-attachments/cft-brief-outline-american-labor-history.pdf?1573677511

Mindful. (n.d.). *How to meditate.* https://www.mindful.org/how-to-meditate/

Misra, S., Cheng, L., Genevie, J., & Yuan, M. (2014). The iphone effect: The quality of in-person social interactions in the presence of mobile devices. *Environment and Behavior, 48*(2), 275-298. 10.1177/0013916514539755

Morris, M. (2011, March 12). A day of rest enters the digital age. *Los Angeles Times.* https://www.latimes.com/local/la-xpm-2011-mar-12-la-me-beliefs-unplugged-20110312-story.html

Nall, R. (2019, April 18). *Does the 20-20-20 rule prevent eye strain?* MedicalNewsToday. https://www.medicalnewstoday.com/articles/321536

National Heart, Lung, and Blood Institute. (n.d.). *How the lungs work.* https://www.nhlbi.nih.gov/health-topics/how-lungs-work

National Institute of General Medical Sciences. (n.d.). *Circadian rhythms.* https://www.nigms.nih.gov/education/fact-sheets/Pages/circadian-rhythms.aspx#:~:text=Circadian%2520rhythms%2520are%2520physical%252C%2520mental,the%2520study%2520of%2520circadian%2520rhythms

National Institute on Aging. (n.d.). *Four types of exercise can improve your health and physical ability.* https://www.nia.nih.gov/health/four-types-exercise-can-improve-your-health-and-physical-ability

Newsom, R. & Rehman, A. (2021, September 20). *Sleep debt and catching up on sleep.* Sleep Foundation. https://www.sleepfoundation.org/how-sleep-works/sleep-debt-and-catch-up-sleep

NHO. (n.d.). *Basics of norwegian labour law.* https://www.nho.no/en/english/articles/basic-labour-law/

Nield, D. (2021, August 30). *Scientists figured out how much exercise you need to 'offset' a day of sitting.* Sciencealert. https://www.sciencealert.com/scientists-figured-out-how-much-exercise-you-need-to-offset-a-day-of-inactivity

Nurit, W. & Avrech Bar, M. (2003). Rest: A qualitative exploration of the phenomenon. *Occupational Therapy International, 10*(4), 227-238. 10.1002/oti.187.

Packer-Kinlaw, D. (2013). *The american dream.* Grey House Publishing. https://www.salempress.com/Media/SalemPress/samples/american_dream_pgs.pdf

Park, W. (2019, December 14). *Should spain replace the siesta with flexible work?* BBC worklife 101. https://www.bbc.com/worklife/article/20191213-should-spain-replace-the-siesta-with-flexible-work

Parker-Pope, T. (n.d.). How to find a hobby. *New York Times.* https://www.nytimes.com/guides/smarterliving/how-to-find-a-hobby

Pew Research Center. (2016, October 6). *The State of American Jobs: How the shifting economic landscape is reshaping work and society and affecting the way people think about the skills and training they need to get ahead.* https://www.pewresearch.org/social-trends/2016/10/06/the-state-of-american-jobs/

Porter, G. (2010). Work ethic and ethical work: Distortions in the american dream. *Journal of Business Ethics, 96*(4), 535–550. http://www.jstor.org/stable/29789736

Powell, A. (2018, April 9). *When science meets mindfulness.* The Harvard Gazette. https://news.harvard.edu/gazette/story/2018/04/harvard-researchers-study-how-mindfulness-may-change-the-brain-in-depressed-patients/

Prelle, M. (2018, September 20). *There's no running in forest bathing.* REI. https://www.rei.com/blog/hike/theres-no-running-in-forest-bathing

Przybylski, A. & Weinstein, N. (2012). Can you connect with me now? How the presence of mobile communication technology influences face-to-face conversation quality. *JSPR, 30*(3), 237-246. 10.1177/0265407512453827

Reissman, H. (2019, February 20). *How to declutter your mind.* Ideas.Ted.Com. https://ideas.ted.com/how-to-declutter-your-mind/

Reynolds, G. (2021, September 15). How much exercise do we need to live longer? *New York Times.* https://www.nytimes.com/2021/09/15/well/move/exercise-daily-steps-recommended.html

Rosario, I. (2020, April 3). *When the 'hustle' isn't enough.* NPR. https://www.npr.org/sections/codeswitch/2020/04/03/826015780/when-the-hustle-isnt-enough

Roth, C. (2011, February 1). *The importance of ergonomics for the safety professional.* EHS Today. https://www.ehstoday.com/archive/article/21912602/the-importance-of-ergonomics-for-the-safety-professional

Salmon, P. (2001). Effects of physical exercise on anxiety, depression, and sensitivity to stress: A unifying theory. *Clinical Psychology Review, 21*(1), 33-61. https://doi.org/10.1016/S0272-7358(99)00032-X

Schatz, K. (2019, February 11). *Your brain on meditation.* Medium. https://medium.com/@kristileeschatz/your-brain-on-meditation-344a63efba73

Senior Lifestyle. (n.d.). *7 best exercises for seniors (and a few to avoid!).* https://www.seniorlifestyle.com/resources/blog/7-best-exercises-for-seniors-and-a-few-to-avoid/

Shibata, M. (2019, August 12). *Why overtired japan is turning to office siestas.* BBC worklife 101. https://www.bbc.com/worklife/article/20190809-why-overtired-japan-is-turning-to-office-siestas

Sianoka, M., Syrek, C., Bloom, J., Korpela, K., & Kinnunen, U. (2018). Enhancing daily well-being at work through lunchtime park walks and relaxation exercises: Recovery experiences as mediators. *Journal of Occupational Health Psychology, 23*(3), 428-442. 10.1037/ocp0000083

Silverton, L. (2020, November 30). *Why the breath is so essential in yoga + 4 yogic breathing techniques.* Mindbodygreen.

https://www.mindbodygreen.com/0-6751/Mastering-the-Full-Yogic-Breath.html

Skilled at Life. (n.d.). *Why hobbies are important.* https://www.skilledatlife.com/why-hobbies-are-important/

Song, C., Ikei, H., & Miyazaki, Y. (2021). Effects of forest-derived visual, auditory, and combined stimuli. *Urban Forestry & Urban Greening, 64,* 127253. https://doi.org/10.1016/j.ufug.2021.127253

Stieg, C. (2020, January 9). *Work-life balance secrets from the happiest countries in the world.* CNBC make it. https://www.cnbc.com/2020/01/09/are-danish-people-really-happy-nordic-work-life-balance-secrets.html

Stress. (2021, September 17). Mental Health Foundation. Retrieved August 30, 2021, from https://www.mentalhealth.org.uk/a-to-z/s/stress

Summer, J. & Vivian, D. (2018). Ecotherapy - a forgotten ecosystem service: A review. *Frontiers in Psychology, 9,* 1389. 10.3389/fpsyg.2018.01389

Sutarto, A., Wahab, M., & Zin, N. (2012). Resonant breathing biofeedback training for stress reduction among manufacturing operators. *Int J Occup Saf Ergon, 18*(4):549-561. 10.1080/10803548.2012.11076959

Suttie, J. (2018, October 29). *5 science-backed reasons mindfulness meditation is good for your health.* Mindful. https://www.mindful.org/five-ways-mindfulness-meditation-is-good-for-your-health/

Taft, M. (2011, September 4). *Downtime for the stone age brain.* Huffpost. https://www.huffpost.com/entry/downtime-for-the-stone-ag_b_889446

The Best of Health. (2020, April 2). *The joy of reading: Is your eReader damaging your eyesight?* https://www.thebestofhealth.co.uk/health-tech/the-joy-of-reading-is-your-ereader-damaging-your-eyesight/

The Conversation. (2021, February 11). *The science behind why hobbies can improve our mental health.* https://theconversation.com/the-science-behind-why-hobbies-can-improve-our-mental-health-153828

Uhls, Y., Michikyan, M., Morris, J., Garcia, D., Small, G., Zgouro, E., & Greenfield, P. (2014). Five days at outdoor education camp without screens improves preteen skills with nonverbal emotion cues. *Computers in Human Behavior 39*(2014), 387-392. http://dx.doi.org/10.1016/j.chb.2014.05.036

U.S. Bureau of Labor Statistics. (2015, June 29). *Time spent in leisure activities in 2014, by gender, age, and educational attainment.* https://www.bls.gov/opub/ted/2015/time-spent-in-leisure-activities-in-2014-by-gender-age-and-educational-attainment.htm

U.S. Bureau of Labor Statistics. (n.d.) *American time use survey.* https://www.bls.gov/tus/

U.S. Department of Labor. (n.d.). *Breaks and meal periods.* https://www.dol.gov/general/topic/workhours/breaks

Van Den Berg, M., Signal, T., & Gander, P. (2019). Fatigue risk management for cabin crew: The importance of company support and sufficient rest for work-life balance-a qualitative study. *Industrial Health, 58*(1), 2-14. https://dx.doi.org/10.2486%2Findhealth.2018-0233

Walker, M. (2017, October 24). *Why your brain needs to dream.* Greater good science center. https://greatergood.berkeley.edu/article/item/why_your_brain_needs_to_dream

Ward, A., Duke, K., Gneezy, A., & Bos, M. (2017). Brain drain: The mere presence of one's own smartphone reduces available cognitive capacity. *Journal of the Association for Consumer Research, 2*(2), 140-154. https://doi.org/10.1086/691462

Ward, M. (2017, August 2). *3 science-backed reasons having a hobby will help your career.* CNBC make it. https://www.cnbc.com/2017/08/02/3-science-backed-reasons-having-a-hobby-will-help-your-career.html

Weir, K. (2019, January). *Give me a break.* American Psychological Association. https://www.apa.org/monitor/2019/01/break

Wetzel, C., Kneebone, R., Woloshynowych, M., Nestel, D., Moorthy, K., Kidd, J., & Darzi, A. (2006). The effects of stress on surgical performance. *The American Journal of Surgery, 191* (1), 5-10. https://doi.org/10.1016/j.amjsurg.2005.08.034

World Health Organization. (2020, November 26). *Physical activity.* https://www.who.int/news-room/fact-sheets/detail/physical-activity

Printed in Great Britain
by Amazon